Nurturing the wellbeing of students in difficulty

Nurturing the wellbeing of students in difficulty

The legacy of Paul Cooper

Carmel Cefai (ed.)

PETER LANG
Oxford · Berlin · Bruxelles · Chennai · Lausanne · New York

Bibliographic information published by the Deutsche Nationalbibliothek.
The German National Library lists this publication in the German National Bibliography;
detailed bibliographic data is available on the Internet at http://dnb.d-nb.de.

A catalogue record for this book is available from the British Library.

Library of Congress Cataloging-in-Publication Data

Names: Cefai, Carmel, editor.
Title: Nurturing the wellbeing of students in difficulty: the legacy of
    Paul Cooper / Edited by Carmel Cefai.
Description: NewYork, NY: PeterLang, [2024] | Includes bibliographical
    references and index.
Identifiers: LCCN 2024011741 | ISBN 9781803743424 (paperback) | ISBN
    9781803743431 (ebook) | ISBN 9781803743448 (epub)
Subjects: LCSH: Students with social disabilities--Education. | Students
    with social disabilities--Mental health. | Social learning. | Emotions
    in children. | Problem children--Behavior modification. | Cooper, Paul,
    1955-.
Classification: LCC LC4065. N87 2024 | DDC 371.826/94--dc23/eng/20240328
LC record available at https://lccn.loc.gov/2024011741

Cover image by Paul Cooper.
Cover design by Peter Lang Group AG

ISBN 978-1-80374-342-4 (print)
ISBN 978-1-80374-343-1 (ePDF)
ISBN 978-1-80374-344-8 (ePub)
DOI 10.3726/b21409

© 2024 Peter Lang Group AG, Lausanne
Published by Peter Lang Ltd, Oxford, United Kingdom
info@peterlang.com - www.peterlang.com

Carmel Cefai has asserted his right under the Copyright, Designs and Patents Act, 1988, to
be identified as Editor of this Work.

All rights reserved.
All parts of this publication are protected by copyright.
Any utilisation outside the strict limits of the copyright law, without the permission of the
publisher, is forbidden and liable to prosecution.
This applies in particular to reproductions, translations, microfilming, and storage and processing in electronic retrieval systems.

This publication has been peer reviewed.

Contents

List of Figures — ix

List of Tables — xi

Foreword — xiii

PART I Introducing Paul Cooper — 1

CARMEL CEFAI
1 Introduction — 3

PAUL COOPER
2 A Brief and Incomplete Account of Some Early Adventures in Education — 13

PART II Diversity and Inclusion — 33

MICHALIS KAKOS AND PAUL COOPER
3 Identity as Difference: On Distinctiveness, Cool and Inclusion — 35

BRAHM NORWICH
4 The Biopsychosocial Model and What It Means for Understanding Inclusion in Education — 53

PAUL DOWNES
5 Reframing Cooper's Emotional-Relational, Commodification and Biopsychosocial Concerns as a Spatial Turn towards Concentric Systems of Inclusion — 67

VALERIA CAVIONI AND GIUSI ANTONIA TOTO
6 Exploring Pre-service Special Education Teachers' Self-
Perceptions in Addressing Students' Academic, Social, and
Emotional Needs   85

SU QIONG XU
7 The Curriculum Reforms of Special Education in the Context
of Inclusive Education in China   109

PART III   Nurture Groups   125

DAVID COLLEY
8 From Nurture Groups to Nurturing Cities:
The Impact of Evidence-Based Research   127

CARMEL BORG
9 Returning from Educational Exile: The School of Barbiana
and Emancipatory Nurture Groups as Projects of Hope and
Possibility   139

CORINNA BARKER AND HELEN COWIE
10 Developmental Effects on the Daughters of
Absent Fathers: The Need for Nurture   153

PART IV   Engaging Students with Social, Emotional and
Behavioural Difficulties   173

KATE WINCHESTER AND CHRIS FORLIN
11 Overcoming Disengagement of Students through an
Arts-Based Programme   175

Contents

COLLEEN MCLAUGHLIN
12 Looking the Wrong Way   197

MARIA POULOU
13 From Students 'without voices' to Students with ... 'low voices'   211

COLEEN GILKES-COLLYMORE AND GARRY HORNBY
14 Exploring the Experiences of Mothers of Children with
    ADHD in the Caribbean   229

Notes on Contributors   245

Index   251

Figures

Figure 4.1.	Factors in interaction in the bio-psycho-social model of ADHD	56
Figure 4.2.	Value bases underlying different research stances	60
Figure 5.1.	Diametric dualism	69
Figure 5.2.	Concentric dualism	69
Figure 6.1.	Self-portrait depicting a teacher's openness, caring and empathy	92
Figure 6.2.	Self-portrait depicting the teacher as a gardener taking care of students' needs	93
Figure 6.3.	Self-portrait depicting the teacher as a lighthouse to supervise and guide the students across age stages in their education	94
Figure 6.4.	Self-portrait depicting the teacher as a compass providing directions to students	95
Figure 6.5.	Self-portrait depicting the teacher holding a magic wand to enhance imagination and spark students' interest and participation	96
Figure 6.6.	Self-portrait depicting the teacher's ability to build an atmosphere of serenity and equity	97
Figure 6.7.	Self-portrait illustrating the teacher as an anchor providing stability and assistance to students	98
Figure 6.8.	Self-portrait depicting the teacher holding a road sign with two possible directions	100
Figure 8.1.	The Six Principles of Nurture (courtesy of nurtureuk)	130
Figure 11.1.	Student engagement framework (Munns, 2021, p. 3)	181

Tables

Table 10.1. Participants' explanations for the absence of the father   158
Table 10.2. Reported ages of participants when father became absent   158
Table 10.3. Themes that emerged from the participants' responses   158

Foreword

I was delighted when I was asked to write a foreword to this book which seeks to recognise and honour the significant impact, the many years of work and research undertaken by Professor Paul Cooper has had in his chosen field.

It would be difficult to overstate the importance of his work and the positive outcome it has had on the education and lives of children and young people experiencing some social, emotional, and behavioural difficulties. As I began to think about what I would write I went to my bookshelves and pulled out some of the texts he has written or edited over the many years he has been trying to ensure that those needs are being met; trying to provide the positive outcomes they need to lead happy and fulfilling lives. Looking at the books reinforced my conclusions that his work and research has been and still is significant.

I first met Paul at the National Council meetings of the Association, now called SEBDA but at that time, AWMC, which were held in the opulent boardrooms at St Thomas' Hospital in London. He took on the editorship of our journal transforming it from a somewhat 'in house' one into the internationally respected 'Emotional and Behavioural Difficulties' journal it is today. He was an active member of the Council, working closely with eminent members such as Robert Laslett and Marion Bennathan. His enthusiasm and work with universities gave opportunities for him to help the Association develop training programmes for members thus providing a more skilled and informed work force.

The theme which runs through his work with children and young people and his many and varied areas of research, is his belief that all children matter, including those who present as a challenge in the settings in which they find themselves. During my years working in this field in the UK, they have been given several 'labels' such as, 'Maladjusted', and, in the early 1980s, 'Emotional and Behavioural Difficulties', then 'Social, Emotional and Behavioural Difficulties' and currently, 'Social Emotional and Mental Health. Although, over the years, the labels may have changed, I am not convinced that the actual needs are fundamentally different. In the book 'The Handbook of Social Emotional and Behavioural Difficulties (2006) his opening chapter 'Setting the Scene' he suggests that 'SEBD are most obvious when they appear in the form of disruptive behaviour in the classroom' (p. 1). Conversations with those currently working in schools for children identified as 'SEMH', suggest that this is still, too often, the case.

Moving onto this book, the table of contents and titles of the chapters serve to evidence the wide areas of research and development he has introduced over his many years of work not only in the UK, but over so many countries It is true to say he has a worldwide reputation. His research covers so many strategies, such as ecosystemic and biopsychosocial approaches; the importance of Nurture and nurture groups; attention deficit hyperactivity disorder (ADHD) to name just some. They can now be found in many CPD courses of study for students working with children presenting with some of the labels referred to earlier.

The wide range of backgrounds, knowledge and experience coming together in the book will make it essential reading for anyone wanting or needing to widen their knowledge and understanding of the needs of children and young people and those working with them.

Joan Pritchard, MEd
President SEBDA

Reference

Hunter-Carsch, M., Tiknaz, Y., Cooper, P., & Sage, R. (2006). *The handbook of social, emotional and behavioural difficulties*. Continuum.

PART I

Introducing Paul Cooper

CARMEL CEFAI

1 Introduction

Thirty years ago, Paul Cooper published his first and highly influential book on students with social, emotional and behaviour difficulties (SEBD), *Effective Schools for Disaffected Students* (Cooper, 1993a). The book presented Paul's research on the views of students who were excluded from school because of their challenging behaviour. It provides the narratives of the students themselves on how they could become engaged in their learning once they feel secure and valued and are provided with opportunities for them to be successful. Paul Cooper was one of the first to give a voice and listening ear to students with challenging behaviour. *Learning from pupils' perspectives* (Cooper, 1993b) and *Pupils as partners* (1996) were another two key papers advocating for students' voices at the time. Paul argued that students should be seen as a source of knowledge and expertise, having unique and inside knowledge of what it is like to be a student in a particular context (Cooper, 1996) (see also Cefai & Cooper, 2010). This contrasts with common practices at the time which tended to punish and exclude such students (see Cooper et al., 1994).

It was during this time in the mid-1990s when working on my Master's dissertation on students with SEBD at the University of Wales (Cefai, 1995) that I first came across Paul Cooper's work. One of the key publications which informed the conceptual framework of my dissertation was the paper by Paul and Graham Upon (1991) evocatively titled *Controlling the urge to control. An ecosystemic approach to problem behaviour in schools*. It was a fresh and innovative approach to the conceptualisation and understanding of students with SEBD, contrasting with the prevalent behaviouristic and classroom management approach at the time (e.g. Canter & Canter, 1992). The ecosystemic perspective shifted the focus from the students and their (mis)behaviour towards the interactional patterns and relationships in the social systems in the lives of the students and how these influenced and shaped their behaviour. Paul was clearly challenging lineal, reductionistic and within-child conceptualisations of challenging behaviour (cf. Elton Report, 1989). He also argued that the needs of all the stakeholders, including those of the students themselves, need to be taken into consideration when addressing the issue. For instance, his well-known book with Jerry Olsen *Dealing with Disruptive Students in the Classroom* (2001) which has been adopted as a textbook in numerous courses in Initial Teacher Education courses, takes a systemic approach to classroom management, with behaviour difficulties seen in a broader context particularly in the systemic interactions between the stakeholders involved, including the relationship between the school and the families.

The ecosystemic approach to SEBD was in a way the forerunner to another major contribution of Paul Cooper in this area. The biopsychosocial approach to individual educational needs and disability provided a broad, multifaceted approach to understanding and supporting students with SEBD, integrating sometimes diametrically opposing views such as biologically determined behaviour and socially constructed behaviour (Cooper, 1997, 2008). The biopsychosocial perspective of ADHD, one of the first to construe ADHD from such a broad, integrated approach, 'was a way to combine and bring together a more complex synthesis not just as an intellectual exercise, but as critical to enhancing educational practice, especially for those with disability and difficulties' (Norwich, this volume). The educational psychology students and learning support educators at the University of Malta had the opportunity to listen directly to Paul explaining how this perspective may be effectively applied to understand and address the needs of students with SEBD such as those manifesting externalising problems, internalising problems, and ADHD (see Part II of this book).

The biopsychosocial perspective was also instrumental 'to expand' how inclusion and inclusive education are construed and understood (Norwich, this volume), steering the narrative away from either/or dichotomous positions. Paul moved away from exclusive ideological positions, promoting instead an evidence-based and 'what works' approach, clearly outlined in his books *We can work it out: What works in educating pupils with social emotional and behavioural difficulties: Inclusive practice in mainstream schools* (Cooper, 2001) and *From inclusion to engagement: Helping students engage with schooling through policy and practice* (Cooper & Jacobs, 2011). This approach is embodied in another major contribution by Paul Cooper, both in the UK and internationally, namely Nurture Groups. Nurture Groups were developed in the UK as an educational provision to support the educational needs of students with social, emotional and behaviour difficulties (Colley, this volume). Paul was instrumental in establishing nurture groups as an innovative, evidence-based practice in the UK and abroad such as Canada and Malta through a series of evaluation studies he carried out with colleagues (Colley, this volume; Cooper et al., 2001; Cooper & Tiknaz, 2005; Cooper & Whitebread, 2007) (see Part III of this book).

Nurture Groups were construed as a short-term programme within mainstream primary schools, providing intensive educational and psychosocial support to students with SEBD to facilitate their inclusion back in their mainstream classroom. They were also intended to have a ripple effect on the whole school, leading to a 'nurturing school' (Bennathan & Boxall, 1996). In our paper *The introduction of nurture groups in Maltese schools: A method of promoting inclusive education* (Cefai & Cooper, 2011, p. 69), we argue that the introduction of Nurture Groups in Malta could help 'to extend the capacity of … schools to become more inclusive, and to develop into resource centres for emotional literacy and parental education' facilitated by a 'recog(nition) that successful educational engagement for pupils with SEBD is a developmental process, and in certain circumstances may require forms of interventions that take place in alternative settings for a particular period of time'.

While Paul Cooper was highly impactful in the UK, he was equally influential in the international field. Following his well-established positions at the Universities of Birmingham, Oxford, Cambridge and Leicester, his research and numerous publications on students with SEBD and Nurture Groups in particular, and as editor of the *Emotional and Behaviour Difficulties* for fourteen years, he become one of the leading international authorities on the wellbeing and education of students with SEBD. He held posts at universities in Hong Kong/China, Japan, Australia, Taiwan, Malta and the USA, and carried out teaching and research in various countries such as Australia, Canada, Hong Kong/China, Lebanon,

Malta[1], and USA. He was co-founder of the *European Network for Social and Emotional Competence* (ENSEC) established in 2008, serving as its joint chair and honorary chair for fifteen years. ENSEC is now a well-established network with hundreds of members providing a platform for researchers and practitioners to share knowledge and develop collaborative projects. In 2015 Paul was awarded the Lifetime Achievement Award by the University of Malta in collaboration with ENSEC. Paul was also founding co-editor of the *International Journal of Emotional Education* for fourteen years, now a well-established indexed international journal. This year happens to be the fifteenth anniversary of the founding of ENSEC and the *International Journal of Emotional Education*.

This book seeks to present a snapshot of some of the major academic achievements of Paul Cooper over his forty-year career, through the lens of those who had the privilege of working with him. It brings together former colleagues from the UK and other parts of the world such as Australia, Bermuda, China, Greece, Ireland, Italy and Malta, whose work was influenced by Paul's innovative frameworks, perspectives, and research. This book presents several chapters related to those areas where Paul's work made a significant impact, such as psycho-educational interventions for students with SEBD, social and emotional education, the voices of students with SEBD, the inclusion of students with SEBD, the biopsychosocial perspective, and nurture groups. It is organised into four parts. Part I introduces Paul Cooper's career and work, while the other three parts address the innovative aspects in his work, namely theoretical reviews and practical applications of his innovative ideas on diversity and inclusion (Part II), nurturing environments for learners with SEBD (Part III); and interventions to engage students with SEBD, including the importance of listening the students' voices (Part IV).

In the second chapter, Paul Cooper takes us through his until now unpublished early experiences (or adventures as he calls them) in education and how these helped to shape his future trajectory in the area of

[1] Together with this author, Paul helped to establish Nurture Groups and Learning Support Zones in Maltese schools, provided extensive in-service training to school staff and other practitioners on supporting students with SEBD and ADHD, and helped to set up the first Master Programme in SEBD at the University of Malta.

SEBD. His childhood working-class environment and his experience as a secondary school A-stream student which forced him to play rugby instead of his favourite soccer (soccer and his favourite Foxes (Leicester City FC) are one of his passions), followed by the mind blowing experience of Hargreaves's incisive work on the negative impact of streaming, and his teaching and researching with students with SEBD, were critical influences which shaped his distinct humanistic approach to understanding and supporting students with SEBD and his aversion to punitive, coercive and blaming approaches. Indeed, his approach to SEBD has been one which seeks to understand the pain underlying each student's cry for help, listening to their voices, and seeking to make their educational experience a positive, engaging and rewarding one.

The second part of the book is dedicated to diversity and inclusion and starts with a chapter written by Paul Cooper himself with Michalis Kakos who worked with Paul for some time at the University of Leicester. Drawing on unpublished qualitative research with two groups of adolescents, the authors discuss at length the relationship between group belonging, inclusion and identity construction. They argue that a framework for the understanding of inclusion and identity based on distinctiveness and difference, apart from being theoretically solid, provides a more authentic portrayal of how adolescents experience and perceive identity and group membership.

Brahm Norwich is a contemporary colleague of Paul Cooper, with a focus on individual educational needs and inclusion. In Chapter 4 he describes how Paul's application of the biopsychosocial perspective to individual educational needs and disability, such as ADHD, helped to broaden the discourse about inclusion, moving away from either/or dichotomies towards an integration of biological, psychological, and social processes, and leading to more meaningful and effective educational practice. In Chapter 5, Paul Downes from Dublin City University, Ireland, examines Cooper's work on social and emotional education, nurture groups, the biopsychosocial perspective and inclusion, within a critical spatial framework. Similarly to Norwich, he proposes a shift from 'diametric frames' of either/or dichotomies and 'splitting cultures', towards an integrative 'spatial turn towards concentric systems of inclusion'.

In Chapter 6, Valeria Cavioni who worked with Paul within the ENSEC Network, present together with Guisi Toto an original study on initial teacher education and inclusive education in Italy. Using visual self-portraits and descriptive adjectives and group discussions, the authors examine how special education pre-service teachers in Italy see themselves as prospective teachers effectively supporting the social and emotional needs of students with individual educational needs. Thematic analysis identified several key educator qualities and capacities which are considered crucial in such contexts, including the provision of a nurturing, inclusive and growth-promoting learning environment adapted to the individual needs of the learners, as well as the need for their own personal self-development and growth as educators. In the last chapter in this part, Su Qiong XU who collaborated with Paul during his term in Hong Kong/China, takes Paul's contributions on individual educational needs and inclusive education to discuss the curriculum reforms of special education and inclusion in China. In her critical analysis of the curricular reform in special education in China, she identifies the challenges in the implementation of an inclusive oriented curriculum and makes various recommendations on how such challenges may be addressed to promote inclusion and equity.

Part III is dedicated to Paul's Cooper pioneering work on Nurture Groups. David Colley, a former PhD student of Paul who continued to work with Paul on evaluating the effectiveness of nurture groups in the UK, opens his chapter with a detailed background of the development and evolution of nurture groups in the UK and their proliferation abroad through Paul Cooper's efforts. He describes how Paul and his colleagues' work on evaluating nurture groups, helped to establish this psycho-educational approach as an innovative, evidence-based intervention for students with SEBD. In Chapter 8, Carmel Borg who collaborated with Paul during his frequent academic visits at the University of Malta, draws on his own work on Don Milani's School of Barbiana in Italy, to propose how nurture groups in Malta may similarly be transformed into emancipatory and liberatory learning support provisions, providing concrete hope and possibility for marginalised children. In the last chapter in this part, Corinna Barker and Helen Cowie, who worked closely with Paul within the ENSEC network, present an original study on the impact of fathers' absence on daughters' social and emotional wellbeing. They explore how nurture groups may operate as an effective intervention for fatherless girls, providing timely and much needed emotional support during the critical school years.

The final part of the book discusses interventions to engage students with SEBD, the centrepiece of Paul Cooper's work. In Chapter 10, Kate Winchester and Chris Forlin who was Paul's colleague during his time at the Institute of Education in Hong Kong/China, present an original study with marginalised children in Australia. They implemented an arts-based programme to help students overcome disengagement, with student feedback indicating that they found that the programme enhanced their social and emotional skills such as risk-taking and empathy as well as their learning engagement. In the following chapter, Colleen McLaughlin, who was Paul Cooper's colleague during his early years at the University of Cambridge, discusses the current situation of out of school children in the UK, the relationship between exclusion and mental health, and how social and emotional education may facilitate engagement, agency, sense of belonging, and connectedness in such children.

Maria Poulou who collaborated with Paul Cooper on several research projects, draws on Paul's seminal work on the importance of listening to the perspectives of students with SEBD, to discuss the current situation of such students in Greece. She concludes that although the voices of these students are now becoming louder, they are still relatively 'low voices' and need to be raised and listened to more carefully by adults. In the final chapter, Coleen Gilkes-Collymore and Garry Hornby, a contemporary colleague of Paul who specialised in inclusive education and psycho-educational interventions for students with individual educational needs, present another original study on the experiences of single mothers of children with ADHD in the Caribbean. They identified the challenges such parents encountered in bringing up their children and in supporting their education, and provided suggestions on how parents may be supported in overcoming such challenges and consequently support their children more effectively.

This book is a recognition of Paul Cooper's extensive work and landmark contributions by some of his previous colleagues and co-researchers. Clearly it is not exhaustive as Paul Cooper's contribution is extensive, multifaceted and spans over 40 years, with over 200 publications and 30 books. It does bring together, however, several colleagues who share some of their important work and insights on how Paul's pioneering work was instrumental in advancing the field they were working on and inspired them to further extend and develop the area themselves. Social, emotional and behaviour difficulties, the perspectives of students with SEBD, nurture groups, the biopsychosocial perspective to individual education needs and disability, the wellbeing of students, especially those most marginalised and disadvantaged, these have become keywords endemically attached to Paul Cooper. Paul Cooper dedicated his academic life researching and writing to advance theory and practice to nurture and enhance the wellbeing of marginalised and disadvantaged children, at a time when such children were not only voiceless and disenfranchised but frequently at the receiving end of punitive, coercive, and exclusionary practices. His work is as relevant today as it was when he started his career forty years ago. Paul Cooper's legacy lives on not only in the extensive work he produced and disseminated, but also in the work he inspired and helped others to achieve. The chapters presented in this book may be seen as another part of this legacy, an important contribution to our understanding of the complex challenges being faced by children and young people today in their education and wellbeing and how these may be effectively addressed.

References

Bennathan, M. & Boxall, M. (1996). *Effective intervention in primary schools: Nurture groups*. David Fulton Publishers.

Canter, L. & Canter, M. (1992). *Assertive discipline: A take charge approach for today's educator*, 2nd edn. Canter & Associates.

Cefai, C. (1995). *Pupils', parents' and teacher's perceptions of behaviour problems and school family interactions in a mainstream primary school*. Unpublished MEd dissertation, University of Wales Swansea.

Cefai, C., & Cooper, P. (2010). Students without voices: The unheard accounts of students with social, emotional and behaviour difficulties. *European Journal of Special Needs Education*, 25(2), 183–198.

Cefai, C., & Cooper, P. (2011). Nurture groups in Maltese schools: Promoting inclusive education. *British Journal of Special Education, 38*(2), 65–72.
Cooper, P. (1993a). *Effective schools for disaffected students*. Routledge.
Cooper, P. (1993b). Learning from pupils' perspectives. *British Journal of Special Education 20*(4), 129–133.
Cooper, P. (1996). Pupils as partners: Pupils' contributions to the governance of schools. In K. Jones & T. Charlton (Eds), *Overcoming learning and behaviour difficulties* (pp. 192–207). Routledge.
Cooper, P. (1997). Biology, behaviour and education: ADHD and the bio-psycho-social perspective. *Educational and Child Psychology, 14*, 31–38.
Cooper, P. (2001). *We can work it out: What works in educating pupils with social emotional and behavioural difficulties: Inclusive practice in mainstream schools*. Routledge/Falmer.
Cooper, P. (2008). Like alligators bobbing for poodles? A critical discussion of education, ADHD and the biopsychosocial perspective. *Journal of Philosophy of Education, 42*. 10.1111/j.1467-9752.2008.00657.x.
Cooper, P., Arnold, R., & Boyd, E. (2001). The effectiveness of nurture groups: preliminary research findings. *British Journal of Special Education, 28*, 160–166.
Cooper, P. & Jacobs, B. (2011). *From inclusion to engagement: Helping students engage with schooling through policy and practice*. Wiley Blackwell.
Cooper, P., Smith, C., & Upton, G. (1994). *Emotional and behaviour difficulties*. Routledge.
Cooper, P., & Tiknaz, Y. (2005). Progress and challenge in nurture groups: Evidence from three case studies. *British Journal of Special Education, 32*, 211–222.
Cooper, P., & Upton, G. (1991). Controlling the urge to control: An ecosystemic approach to problem behaviour in schools. *SfL, 6*(1), 22–26.
Cooper, P., & Whitebread, D. (2007). The effectiveness of nurture groups on student progress: Evidence from a national research study. *Emotional and Behavioural Difficulties, 12*. 10.1080/13632750701489915.
Elton Report. (1989). *Discipline in schools*. DES.
Olsen, J., & Cooper, P. (2001). *Dealing with disruptive students in the classroom*. Routledge.

PAUL COOPER

2 A Brief and Incomplete Account of Some Early Adventures in Education

In the Beginning

I was born into a working-class family[1] in the late December 1955. At that time my mum was a full-time housewife (as they called them then) and my dad was a carpenter. I had two older brothers, one eight and one six years older than me. My parents were what might now be called 'upwardly mobile'. They aspired to home ownership and abandoned their brand new, bright, and shiny council house with indoor facilities for a dark Victorian mid terrace with outside toilet. But this was a 'private' house, as they used to say. It cost all of £800 (that's about £17k in 2023 – these houses sell for £200,000 these days). The point is that I grew up in a family that was relatively financially poor, but aspirational. I was also the late addition which meant that later I became an only child when my brothers left home – one at age 16 and the other at age 15. The good news was that by this time we had a new house with indoor plumbing.

---

1 On social class: when I applied for university in 1973 my father's occupation as entered on my UCCA form was 'RAF NCO/Airframe Fitter'. By the time I married in 1980, he was recorded on our wedding certificate as a 'Civil Servant'. He had taken advantage of educational opportunities available to RAF personnel in those days, and when he retired from the RAF, age 55, he secured an administrative post with the Manpower Services Commission, which meant that he (by some definitions) ascended to the middle class. He hated that job, because it bored him to death, and he had no interest in social class – his or anyone else's. This said, he probably lived quite a bit longer than if after his first retirement he had returned to working on building sites.

In those days most people still had, like us, coal or coke fuelled open fires in their living rooms. Added to the fact that everyone (it seemed) smoked tobacco in those days, it's no surprise that I inherited a family weakness on for bronchitis, which meant that I missed significant amounts of my primary school education. To cut to the chase: I had a lot of scope in my primary school years for autodidacticism, which turned out to be a good training for self-directed learning in school and beyond. I had the advantage of having access to my eldest brother's *'Look and Learn'* magazines, which he had collected between 1962 and 1964, as well as a decent local public library, and my parents' eclectic book collection. I failed the 11+ but had the luck to be in the catchment area of a very good secondary modern school. I say 'very good' but not for everyone (see below). I did well in secondary school as my health improved. I achieved 9 O levels and went on to a sixth form in a grammar school where I qualified for a place at university. Like a lot of people in those days I was the first in my family to achieve this. This would never have happened with the support of my brilliant A level English teacher, Mrs Sandra Hopkins.

I feel that my then apparently slightly atypical route to university and an academic career provided me with insights that I might not otherwise have had, and I have no doubt that this influenced my choice of career and issues I chose to focus on in my research.

Learning to Study Education

My major at Stirling University was English Studies (1974–1978). The course I chose lasted 4.5 years and involved taking a Diploma in Education (with QTS) concurrently with my degree between the second and final years. This meant that from the second year onwards I was studying the sociology, psychology and philosophy of education and becoming acquainted with key educational issues, controversies, and debates of the time. I was also able to devote one third of my time in the first year to the study of philosophy and one third to sociology, alongside English literature. I now think that this combination of subjects was very useful foundation for my future academic career. The contribution of groundings in philosophy and sociology to the mental equipment of an academic educationist should be obvious, but for me of equal importance were the skills of textual analysis that I acquired through my studies of literary texts. I recently calculated that over the course of my degree I wrote over 50,000 words for courses in the English strand alone, much of this was devoted to close textual analysis. The constant requirement to produce essays of between 1,500 and 6,000 words, plus a 15–20,000 final dissertation were a good preparation for the 'publish or perish', research-focused world of academia where I went on to make a living.

The first full blown 'Education' book I recall reading was David Hargreaves's (1967) *Social Relations in a Secondary School*. As an aspiring literary scholar, I was a bit snooty about the idea of any book about schools and teaching, or any book, for that matter (I sometimes suspect), written by anyone who was still alive. I was deeply underwhelmed by the title and decided that this was going to be such a dull read that I'd 'skim' it – a technique well known to undergraduates (and too many professors, I suspect) that involves reading the bits of the introduction and most of the conclusion, and then using the index to sample the text in between. From the moment I opened that Hargreaves book I was drawn in by a compelling writing style and a piercing analysis of the educational challenges faced by working class pupils at that time. I believe that, though the specifics are different, the basic message is as valid now as it was then. Hargreaves's reliance on the first-hand testimony of students, and his sensitive interpretations of that testimony are masterful. At the centre of this excellent book is an evidence-based condemnation of the streaming system that was prevalent in schools in those days.

Hargreaves's book resonated with my experience in ways I did not expect. 'Lumley School' (the pseudonym Hargreaves used for the school that was the site for his research) echoed many features of the secondary that I had attended. Both Lumley Secondary and my school were boys' only schools and had rigid streaming systems, Lumley's went from A to D over the four compulsory years of secondary education. My school's streaming system went from A to E for the first three years. In Year 4 the streams were further divided into two 'Certificate' streams and three 'Leavers'' streams. Obviously, in fifth year only student from the 'Certificate' streams remained.

My personal experience echoed Hargreaves's finding that the stream students entered at age 11, for most students, was the one they would most likely still be in at their point of exit four or five years later. Limited opportunities were created to enable mobility between streams in the form of annual promotions and demotions for a few students in each form, but for most students the designation of being an A, B, C, D or E student became an important signifier of academic and social status.

Hargreaves adopted a Symbolic Interactionist approach (Mead, 1934; Blumer, 1986) in his study, which emphasises the ways in which human beings' sense of reality is a product of the subjective meanings they attach to elements in their environment. These meanings are influenced strongly by values, beliefs and symbols that are developed and passed on through social interaction (Sleeves, 2023). It follows that empirical research based on this approach must rely heavily on the subjective experience of participants in the social setting that is being studied using ethnographic methods pioneered in social anthropology. As a result of this approach, conventional wisdom at that time about the efficacy of streaming was confounded. The most striking finding was that there was a direct relationship between stream placement and commitment to the espoused values of the school: the lower the stream the less inclined students were to be supportive of the values of the school. The reasons for this association, revealed in the students' accounts, were that higher stream pupils tended to be motivated by their placement, whilst lower stream pupils were de-motivated and increasingly alienated from the school and its espoused values. The system that was intended to foster and support educational opportunities in relation to students' aptitudes and abilities benefitted only the students at top of the hierarchy, leaving the lower stream students with a sense of being under-valued and marginalised.

Social Relations in a Secondary School is probably the single most important influence on my desire to become a teacher and then an educational researcher. It did for me what a good piece of research should do, it made me see aspects of my world in a new way. It made me realise that my secondary education had been characterised by a pattern of segregation and privilege. Students in the A and B streams had a completely different school experience to those in the C, D and E streams. We were taught exclusively by the senior staff (including the headmaster and deputy headmaster); the other streams were catered for by a group of staff who we knew by name but who were never assigned to teach us. The only times we did come across them were in extra-curricular contexts, such as the preparations for the annual school dramatic production, and the annual youth hostelling trip to Wales (activities that were not particularly popular with students from the lower streams). This did not include extra-curricular sports: the A and B streams had to do rugby in our games' lessons, whilst the C, D and E streams did football (i.e. soccer). This meant that the school rugby teams that represented the school in competitions with other schools were selected only from boys in the A and B streams, and the soccer teams from the lower streams (a rare advantage for lower stream boys, though even then some higher stream boys got into these teams through the provision of open 'trials' that were held annually). And, of course, when it came to the selection of prefects, these were drawn exclusively from the A and B streams in the fifth year from which the lower streams were excluded because they did not exist after the fourth year. It is with dry amusement that I recall the epiphany that I experienced as I digested David Hargreaves's book. I remember realising for the first time: 'so that's why they hate us!' It had always been a mystery to me why some of the kids in the lower streams took such exception to the kids in A stream. I remember finding myself with friends (also A streamers) being confronted in the street and, on at least one occasion, being chased with threats of fatal violence by a group of fellow pupils, none of whom any of us knew by name, but who we knew to be from C and D streams.

Towards the end of the teacher training element of my course at Stirling University in Scotland, I got to read *Deviance in Classrooms* (Hargreaves et al., 1975), which is another seminal text that provides a fascinating account of how schools can sometimes socially construct pupil deviance. The book was again based on a symbolic interactionist research study. The book charts with forensic detail the ways in which students in the study were, in modern parlance, 'groomed' to be deviant by their teachers through a series of self-fulfilling prophecies. Teacher expectations that certain students were likely to be deviant were established very early on in students' secondary school careers often based on arbitrary cues, such as a child being the younger sibling of a student deemed to be deviant. As time passed, evidence that supported those initial speculations was favoured over evidence that might challenge them. It worked the other way too. Kids whose 'type' was initially assumed to be 'non-deviant' were far more likely to be given the benefit of the doubt when behaving in ways that were deemed to reinforce the deviant identities of other students.

Hargreaves's work sat within a university Education curriculum that emphasised the social context of learning and the importance of interpersonal relations in a student-centred constructivist pedagogy. In addition to this formulation, my arts background led me to discern within this social-constructivist paradigm a key role for the emotional dimension. It was also clear to me from my reading of A. S. Neill (1968) and other radical educationists (e.g. Holt, 1969, 1970; Willis, 1978), as well as from my background in the arts, that the forces of social stratification, labelling and, acceptance and rejection not only produced rational responses in students, but that these rational responses, in essence being accepted or rejected, automatically gave way to *feelings* along a continuum from belonging to alienation, and that this emotional dimension was of central importance in the development of school students' internalised school specific identities.

Such was my formative education in the study of Education, and, in many respects, this is still at the core of how I understand the nature of schooling and its challenges. And I am profoundly grateful to the staff at Stirling University and in the schools where I did numerous teaching practices (see below for more on this) for furnishing with me with what I consider to be an outstanding introduction to the field of study that I would follow for all my working life. This said, the foundations at this point still required further strengthening as the following sections will show.

Becoming a Teacher

There is no doubt in my mind that the study of Education has to include first-hand experience of the particular sphere of education that is the focus of study. Fortunately, in this regard, most of education academics have been school students for at least ten years before we get to university, and this is an important source of understanding from the pupil/student perspective. Of course, our experience of being pupils/students can vary widely. It was common in the 1970s for teacher training students to have had relatively successful school careers. Those who had been to selective secondary schools, had often attended grammar schools. Exceptions to this tended to be mature students who had studied for university entrance qualifications at Further Education colleges. I sometimes think that this might have been the reason why Hargreaves's (1967) *Social Relations in a Secondary School* was a key text on the Education introductory course at Stirling. As I have suggested, the book pulls no punches in relations to the damage that schools can inflict on student aspiration and motivation to engage with the educational process, and as I was to discover subsequently, there are many other empirically based book-length studies that echo and expand on Hargreaves's pioneering work (e.g. Willis, 1978; Ball, 1981; Schostak, 1982; Tattum, 1982; Lawrence et al., 1984; Kronk, 1987).

At Stirling we had annual doses of Teaching Practice (TP), though so as not to interfere with our academic education these always took place in lengths of two, four and six weeks usually in the winter vacation. Only in the final semester in year five did we have a TP in term time. We also had courses of Micro-Teaching, at various points throughout the programme. These were short video-taped sessions in which individual students practised specific teaching skills (e.g. questioning; active listening) with a small group of pupils. The recordings were then used as the basis for one-to-one debriefs with a tutor. There is nothing like real-life experience to help put the ideals of the university classroom into perspective. But if TP was hard (and it was), at least we had some insight into why it was hard which went well beyond 'blaming the kids'.

My four-and-a-half-year degree plus teaching Diploma ended in December 1978 and I took up my first teaching post as an Assistant Teacher of English in an Inner-City Comprehensive school in the East of Scotland. I can't say that I enjoyed the experience, and I can't say that I was particularly good at the job, though I passed my compulsory two-year probation and discovered that I wasn't bad at teaching literature, especially poetry, and stimulating the creativity of students, especially the writing of stories and poetry.

Like most Newly Qualified Teachers (NQTs), especially those who found themselves in 'challenging' schools, I found 'discipline' to be a difficult area to master. Though, in hindsight, I think I made far too much of this at the time and allowed it to overshadow the more positive aspects of my experience as a teacher. In fact, as I recall, most of the time my lessons went well. When I experienced 'discipline problems', these tended to be with a few individuals, rather than groups or whole classes. Also, I had learnt enough from my university course and through practice to try to avoid provoking those pupils with whom I had difficulties, and whilst trying to maintain firm boundaries, I always tried to preempt learning problems and find opportunities for 'catching them being good', as Colin Smith, my main PhD supervisor (a very wise and patient man) would later write (Smith, 1992).

Becoming an Education Academic and Researcher

Before I completed my first year as a qualified teacher, I enrolled on the MEd programme (part-time) at Dundee University. I had two main motivations for this: first, to strengthen my knowledge of educational and psychological theory (the programme was accredited by the British Psychological Society), and second, to do some original research in the form of a 20,000-word research-based dissertation (in addition the completion of ten taught courses, including ones on qualitative and quantitative research methods).

I found this a deeply stimulating and thoroughly rewarding course of study. It was whilst at Dundee that I first became acquainted with Vygotsky's (e.g. Vygotsky, 1978) and Bruner's socio-cultural theories of cognitive development (e.g. Bruner, 1966). My introduction to these giants of twentieth century developmental psychology came first via Douglas Barnes's (1976) work, which is based on empirical research carried out in UK classrooms into the ways in which student-led dialogue in small group settings can promote sometimes startling learning outcomes. This built on work he had carried with Harold Rosen and James Britton (Barnes et al., 1969) which I had been introduced to in my undergraduate studies. Barnes elucidates insights developed by Vygotsky and Bruner, independently of each other, of the central importance of the sharing of intersubjectivities in oral communication as a basis for what Bruner calls the process of 'making sense' of the world. From an educational point of view, this major insight places the learner in the role of an active participant at the heart of the learning process. This was a radical challenge to the traditional portrayal of the student as the passive recipient of knowledge that is transmitted by an adult authority. This is not to say that the teacher has no role in students' cognitive development. Vygotsky describes how the teacher can act as a facilitator of student learning by operating within the individual student's Zone of Proximal Development (ZPD), just as students operate within one another's ZPDs. The more the teacher understands about the child's ZPD (i.e. the space between what they know now, and what they might be able to learn from the base of their current understanding) the more the teacher is able to 'scaffold' the child's movement from what they understand now to new understandings.

Barnes (1976) draws an important distinction between what he terms 'School Knowledge' and 'Action Knowledge'. The former is knowledge that students acquire through being told it as a requirement of the school curriculum; the latter is knowledge that the learner has acquired by asking questions that lead to the discovery of information that they can assimilate into their 'inner map of reality on which [their] actions are based' (Barnes, 1976, p. 80). Action Knowledge is knowledge that is relevant to the individual's actual purposes in life. Of course, if one's purposes include the desire to do well in school and pass exams, then school knowledge has its value. But then, as we all know, the retention of such knowledge tends to be of limited duration once the exam has been sat.

This insight helped me to understand why it is that schools are sometimes so much more effective in getting students to internalise 'the hidden curriculum' (Jackson, 1968), which is so important in the lives of students who become disaffected and who rebel, than the formal curriculum, which these students tend to reject. A key aspect of Action Knowledge is how it relates to one's sense of identity: we need to know and understand certain things to be the kind of person and live the kind of life we want, and to avoid the kinds of identities and lives we don't want (see Willis, 1978). Students (and people in general) who find themselves in situations where they are marginalised and alienated will learn strategies to avoid or stand up against those situations.

Space prevents me from going into more detail in relation to these theoretical influences on my thinking, but these influences were and are profound, not least in terms of what I wanted to research and how I wanted to research it. My understanding of social and psychological processes in relation to education led me of two conclusions:

1. The plight of students who are failed and rejected by education systems was (is) a crucial but neglected priority of those who preside over and run educational systems and institutions.
2. One of the best ways to understand and find pathways to bringing positive change (in relation to #1) was (is) to develop understandings of systems and institutions informed by the perceptions of the people who have aversive experiences of those systems and institutions.

My MEd dissertation (Cooper, 1983) was based on a study of the occupational aspirations of students in a co-ed comprehensive school in a deprived inner-city area. My participants were over eighty students, and my research approach involved eliciting their perceptions using a semi structured essay format that asked open questions about how they imagined their future experiences in the workplace. In that location in those days there was a very low unemployment rate. The students were not primed in any way, rather the essays were written outside of normal lesson time, by students who participated voluntarily. The only information they were given prior to writing these essays was that they were part of a research project by a fellow MEd student of the teacher who administered the data gathering.

The findings indicated that virtually all participants expected to work in unskilled, low or semi-skilled jobs. Interestingly, a large proportion of participants expressed some level of expected alienation from the work setting, and a predominantly instrumental attitude towards their work. The absence of aspirations beyond those that might be expected for that neighbourhood was, on the one hand, unsurprising, but what was also surprising was that there was virtually no evidence of these aspirations being modified by the pupils' experience of schooling. The analysis found that these outcomes were consistent with existing theories concerning social and cultural reproduction and the role of schools in supporting as opposed to challenging these processes (cf. Willis, 1978; Harris, 1979; Schostak, 1982; Hargreaves, 1967, 1972, 1975, see above).

After completing my MEd I was employed as the sole researcher on a community project exploring the perceptions and needs of unemployed young people living in a small market town close to Dundee (Cooper, 1983b). I then secured a teaching position at a residential school for boys (9–16 years old) with emotional and behavioural difficulties (EBD) in England where I was a class teacher and oversaw the English curriculum. As I have already indicated, my interest in the literature on EBD in schools was by this time well established and I developed this through further reading in the area. I further supplemented this by getting acquainted with literature on different types of educational provision for EBD, especially in relation to residential provision. One of the first books I read in this area was *Pioneer Work with Maladjusted Children* (Bridgeland, 1971). This wide ranging, extensively researched, magisterial book should still, in my view, be on reading lists for students of education. For me the most compelling parts of the book are the accounts of therapeutic communities created by the 'pioneers' of the title. I was deeply impressed by Bridgeland's overview and plunged headlong into tracking down the original writings by some of the pioneers themselves (including Wills, 1941, 1945, 1960; Shaw, 1955; Lyward, 1958, as well as Burn's (1956) first-hand account of Lyward's work at

Finchden Manor School). I was already acquainted with the writing of AS Neill about Summerhill Schools (1968) (see above), but reading Bridgeland led me to Neill's other writings, including a book based on diary charting his early experiences as a state school teacher (Neill, 1916) in which he deplores the use of 'the tawse' (a leather strap that was widely used by teachers in Scottish schools until 1986 when UK law made it illegal for state school staff to inflict corporal punishment on students).

It is true to say that many of these pioneers were influenced by psychodynamic theories and practices in which many of them were trained, and this may seem outdated to many people nowadays. However, the pioneers by and large did not employ psychoanalysis (Dawson, 1981), rather they used psychoanalytic principles in their day-to-day practise, including:

1. The showing of unconditional positive regard towards students.
2. The sanctioning of 'acting out' by students, whereby repressed, hostile feelings could be express.
3. The encouragement of student autonomy through the practise of 'shared responsibility' (Wills, 1960) among students.
4. The use psychodynamic interpretations of challenging behaviour (i.e.: seeing challenging behaviour as an expression of unmet need, as opposed to being something needing to be repressed through punishment).
(based on Dawson, 1980)

In much the same way as modern-day Nurture Groups (Bennathan and Boxall, 1996) are sometimes (though not always) claimed to draw on Bowlby's (1969) Attachment Theory, in practice, when they work well, they apply the positive principles of AT in their pedagogy and avoid the potentially pathologising aspects of AT which have sometimes been associated a 'blame the parents' approach.

I learned something about practicality from studying the pioneers, and as a result in my second year in post was supported by the school when I initiated a Home Economics strand to the curriculum at the school, as well as initiating the more obvious thing for an English teacher of creating a school magazine and organising 'the school drama production'. I was also the goalkeeper for the staff five-aside football team. This may not be relevant, but for me it was slight bonus for having been forced to play rugby in my secondary school days, because to play rugby to a reasonable standard you need to know how to catch and hold a ball.

A year into my time at the school I enrolled for a PhD at Birmingham University. The chair of my interview panel was the late Professor Ron Gulliford, who remains a major figure in the development of the academic study of what was then called 'Special Education' (Birmingham was the first UK university to appoint a professor of SEN, and Ron Gulliford was the first appointee). My PhD (Cooper, 1989) focused on the effects of residential schooling on students with EBD and their perceptions of the quality of their experience. It was an ethnographic study and was heavily influenced by Hargreaves (1967 – see above), though my methodology was influenced by recent developments in the field (e.g. Hammersley and Atkinson, 1983). I studied two schools, one of which I worked in at the time. It was important to have a second school as a comparison. In addition to one-to-one informant style interviews (Powney & Watts, 1987) with students (n = 28), staff were also interviewed, and a questionnaire was devised (based on findings from the interviews) to ascertain views of students who were not interviewed. In the end data was gathered from a total of fifty-seven students out of a total of seventy-seven across both schools, giving an overall participation rate of 74%. Interviews were also carried with a small number of staff (n = 14) for purposes of triangulation.

The major findings of the study were that, whilst there was some evidence of homesickness and concerns about lack of contact with family (especially in one of the schools which had for provision for fifty-two-week placements and opposed term time only in the other school) there was an overwhelming sense of positivity expressed by participants about the residential experience. Three main aspects of this positivity were:

1. The residential environment provided *respite* from negative experiences in their home/family neighbourhood settings, such as: relationship problems with family members; negative economic circumstances at home; negative experiences of mainstream school

in the form poor relationships with staff and/or fellow pupils, and the influence of delinquent peers.
2. The residential environment provided high quality *relationships*, particularly with teaching and care staff who were characterised a caring, supportive, and willing to listen to students' points of view in ways that had been extremely rare in their mainstream school. Participants talked about the ways in which teaching staff in these schools were more attentive to their learning needs than those in 'ordinary schools' had been. Students felt that they had particular members of staff to whom they could go when they experienced emotional upsets and other personal issues.
3. The majority of students who were well established in both schools held the belief that the schools provided them with opportunities to shed negative labels they had acquired in their earlier educational careers and to internalise more positive images of themselves as possessors of valuable qualities and positive potential. This process is summarised in the term *Re-Signification* and was achieved through supportive relationships with staff (see above) as well as the provision of opportunities to achieve success across a range of activities including personal, social, and academic progress; mastering new skills; participation in group decision making in relation to defined areas of school activity.

Although these schools could be termed to a greater or lesser degree 'total institutions' (TI), the experience of most students in this study did not reflect the patterns of institutionalisation, dehumanisation and abuse that Goffman (1961) identified in his study of TIs. In fact, participants were more likely to attribute those kinds of effects to mainstream schools that they had attended: schools, that had ultimately rejected them and set them on pathways leading to their placement in a residential school.

This is not to say that these findings apply to all residential schools of this type. This study provides a snapshot of two schools at a particular time. What these schools were like before and after the study took place, and what earlier and later groups of students thought of their experiences may be very different from what was shown here. There is no doubt that residential care for children has come in for a lot of criticism since I carried out this study. All I can say is that this is what I found when I engaged in a systematic investigation into what the students in these schools thought about their experience, and how their experience sat in relation to their internal worlds that were informed by earlier and wider experiences.

When, a while later, I decided to turn my PhD thesis into my first book exactly thirty years ago (Cooper, 1993), I decided to consider my original study in the light of school effectiveness theory (e.g. Rutter et al., 1979; Mortimore et al., 1988; Reynolds, 1985). I tracked down what was at the time a much lauded 'effective comprehensive school' that was being heralded for the excellent work it was doing in an area of high social deprivation. I carried out informant style (see above) interviews with a teaching staff, the head teacher, and a group of randomly selected students. I found ample evidence that students in the school felt valued by staff and saw the school as a positive place to be, and for some it was a kind of haven (cf. *Respite*); they enjoyed positive and supportive *relationships* with staff (which included a school counsellor) at all levels, and they believed the school to be a place where they could flourish in ways that would lead on to improved life chances (cf. *re-signification*). The staff expressed values consistent with these student experiences. I felt that this showed that there were ways in which mainstream schools could achieve similar outcomes for students as those I had found in the residential study. However, there continues to be evidence all around us that nowhere near enough mainstream schools are successful in this way, as is demonstrated by the continuing problems of school exclusion, unmet mental health needs in schools, and the ongoing, seemingly relentless stranglehold that social deprivation has on educational engagement and academic achievement (e.g. Crenner-Jennings, 2018). This leads me to conclude that we need to make available the best examples of educational provision available, regardless of the mainstream/specialist divide. There is no room for blind dogma or unflinching, unexamined ideology in the field of education, especially in relation to the education of our most vulnerable children and young people.

Beyond Schools

Before completing my PhD, I left the residential school and went to work briefly in an inner-city Educational Guidance Centre as a class teacher and tutor in English and Maths. This was a day facility for excluded students of secondary school age. I could not help thinking how these students might have benefited from their time in one of the residential schools that I had recently studied. Attendance at the centre was erratic, and there was a sense of defeat pervading the semi-derelict Victorian primary school building where the centre was housed. The sense of hopelessness and professional impotence that went with it made this the most stressful period of my teaching career, and I lasted less than a year, choosing to devote myself to completing my thesis full-time.

It wasn't long, however, before I felt the need to return to the classroom, and at the beginning of the following academic year I took up the post of a Year 5 teacher in a county junior school. I went on to enjoy two of the most enjoyable and rewarding years in my school teaching career. The school was the only one to cater for the junior school aged population of the town it served, so it was truly comprehensive in its intake. Although it was (is) a prosperous town, it was (is) located in a sparsely populated county and the town itself contained at least one pocket that experienced 'rural deprivation'. This said, the school was well run by a dedicated and caring staff and my first class of thirty 9–10 year olds was a delight to work with. These children were cheerful, friendly, and enthusiastic about almost *everything*. The only limiting factor was my imagination. The following year's class was equally delightful.

When it finally came time for me to leave that school I was conflicted, but a research fellowship in EBD had come up at Birmingham University School of Education, where I was studying for my doctorate, and I felt compelled to apply for it. I got the job and in June 1989 I embarked on a study of applications of family therapy theory and techniques to EBD in schools, under Professor Graham Upton. I completed my PhD in my first term there and went on to write and subsequently publish my first book (Cooper, 1993). I also started to in write my second book with Graham and Colin Smith (Cooper et al., 1994), who had been my main doctoral supervisor.

In both its school and university sectors, the educational world contains some of the most decent, civilised, caring, and generous people, you could ever want to meet. Sadly, there a few people in this world devoted to improving the conditions and opportunities of all learners who are not decent, civilised, caring and generous, and I have had the misfortune to meet a few of these. There is no place in education institutions for staff who are uncaring, narcissistic, bullying, dismissive, judgemental, and manipulative, but they are there. Fortunately for me, the people who have been positive influences on me and my early and later career, are of the former type. Like all good teachers they were gentle guides, honest but caring critics and, above all, people of the highest ability and integrity. I can only thank them for helping in what has been for me a most enjoyable and rewarding career. If I were to continue the story into my later career there would be many more people to acknowledge and thank. But as is often the case in academia, I have a word limit that I have already exceeded.

Thanks

Before I end this chapter, I must thank all the colleagues who have contributed to this volume and to Carmel Cefai for initiating and organising its production. As Carmel has stated in his introduction, we've done a great deal of work together in Malta in relation to SEBD in schools, and in the founding of ENSEC and *The International Journal of Emotional Education*. I cherish memories of the warmth and generosity of the welcome I received in Malta, and I am proud of the work we did with the help of several of his colleagues.

All the contributors in this edition are people with whom I have worked either in direct collaboration in research and writing projects, through my work with ENSEC, and/or through my editorial work with *The International Journal of Emotional Education*, and *Emotional and Behavioural Difficulties* (the SEBDA journal).

I would also like to mention some people who are sadly no longer with us, but who were extremely important to me in my professional/academic development, and to whom I am eternally grateful. They include Robert Laslett (Birmingham University), Donald McIntyre (Stirling, Oxford and Cambridge Universities), Jane Lovey (Cambridge University), Marion Bennathan (AWMC/SEBDA) and Stella Chong (Hong Kong Institute of Education). These are people I encountered at different phases of my career from whom I benefited because of their humanity, expertise, generosity, and wisdom. I can think of no better real-life exemplars of some of the themes that have been discussed in the preceding sections.

Finally ...

I thought I might end on a light but at the same time pertinent note. Just in case anyone who reads this chapter, but not very carefully, gets the wrong end of the stick, and decides to threaten me with court action (yes, it did happen once!), please note the following review that I found recently (02 09 23) on local supermarket website:

Linda McCartney's <u>Vegetarian</u> *Hoisin Duck Bites.*   <u>Meat free</u> *pioneer since 1991.*   <u>Vegetarian Society Vegan Approved</u>.   One reviewer (F1Moose – must be a man) gives the product **one star (out of five)**, complaining (capitalization as in the original):   *'Misleading title:*   *Doesn't contain Duck, even though it says so.'*   [PC: It seems we educationists and educators still have a lot of work to do ...]

References

Ball, S. (1981). *Beachside comprehensive*. Cambridge University Press.
Barnes, D. (1976). *From communication to curriculum*. Penguin.
Barnes, D., Britton, J. & Rosen, H. (1969). *Language, the learner, and the school*. Penguin.
Bennathan, M. & Boxall, J. (1996). *Effective intervention in primary schools: Nurture groups*. David Fulton.
Blumer, H. (1986). *Symbolic interactionism: Perspective and method*. University of California Press.
Bowlby, J. (1969). *Attachment: Attachment and loss* (Vol. 1). Basic Books.
Bridgeland, M. (1971). *Pioneer work with Maladjusted children: A study of the development of therapeutic education*. Staples Press.
Bruner, J. (1966). *Towards a theory of instruction*. Harvard University Press.
Burn, M. (1956). *Mr Lyward's answer*. Hamish Hamilton.
Cooper, P. (1983a). *Ideology, education and work: 'A study of the effects of ideology on school pupils' attitudes to the adult world of work.'* Dissertation submitted in partial fulfilment of the requirements for the degree of MEd, University of Dundee.
Cooper, P. (1983b). *The needs and circumstances of unemployed persons between the ages of 16 and 21, living in the Blairgowrie area*. Blairgowrie: The Blairgowrie Youth Project (Unpublished research report).
Cooper, P. (1989). *Respite, relationships and re-signification: A study of the effects of residential schooling on children with emotional and behavioural difficulties, with particular reference to the pupils' perspective*, PhD thesis, University of Birmingham.
Cooper, P. (1993). *Effective schools for disaffected students*. Routledge.
Cooper, P., Smith, C. J. & Upton, G. (1994). *Emotional and behavioural difficulties: Theory to practice*. Routledge.
Crenner-Jennings, W. (2018). *Key drivers of the disadvantage gap literature review: Education in England annual report*, Education Policy Institute <https://epi.org.uk/wp-content/uploads/2018/07/EPI-Annual-Report-2018-Lit-review.pdf>
Dawson, R. (1980). The place of four pioneer tenets in modern practice and opinion. *New Growth*, *1*(2), 44–47.
Goffman, E. (1961). *Asylums*. Penguin.
Hammersley, M. & Atkinson, P. (1983). *Ethnography: Principles in practice*. Routledge.

Hargreaves, D. (1967). *Social relations in a secondary school.* Routledge, Kegan-Paul.
Hargreaves, D. H. (1972). *Interpersonal relations and education.* Routledge, Kegan Paul.
Hargreaves, D., Hester, S. & Mellor, F. (1975). *Deviance in classrooms.* Routledge, Kegan-Paul.
Harris, K. (1979). *Education and knowledge: The structured misrepresentation of reality.* Routledge, Kegan-Paul.
Holt, J. (1969). *How children fail.* Penguin.
Holt, J. (1970). *How children learn.* Penguin.
Jackson, P. W. (1968). *Life in classrooms.* Holt, Rinehart, & Winston.
Kronk, K. (1987). *Teacher-pupil conflict in secondary schools.* Falmer.
Lawrence, J., Steed, D. & Young, P. (1984). *Disruptive children-disruptive schools?* Croom-Helm.
Lyward, G. (1958). *The residential care of disturbed children.* NAMH.
Mead, G. H. (1934). *Mind, self, and society.* University of Chicago Press.
Mortimore, P., Sammons, P., Stoll, L., Lewis, D. & Ecob, R. (1988). *School matters: The junior years.* Open Books.
Neill, A. S. (1916). *A Dominie's log.* Herbert Jenkins.
Neill, A. S. (1968). *Summerhill.* Penguin.
Powney, J. & Watts, M. (1987). *Interviewing in educational research.* Routledge.
Reynolds, D. (1985). *Studying school effectiveness.* Falmer.
Rutter, M., Maughan, B., Mortimore, P. & Ouston, J. (1979). *Fifteen thousand hours: Secondary schools and their effects on children.* Open Books.
Schostak, J. (1982). *Maladjusted schooling: Social control and individuality in secondary schooling.* Falmer.
Shaw, O. (1965). *Maladjusted boys.* Allen and Unwin.
Smith, C. J. (1992). Keeping them clever, preventing learning difficulties from becoming behaviour problems. In K. Wheldall (Ed.), *Discipline in schools: Psychological perspective on the Elton report* (pp. 28–35). Routledge.
Steeves, K. (2023). Symbolic interactionism. In J. M. Okoko, S. Tunison & K. D. Walker (Eds), *Varieties of qualitative research methods* (pp. 457–462). Springer texts in education. Cham: Springer. <https://doi.org/10.1007/978-3-031-04394-9_71>
Tattum, D. (1982). *Disruptive pupils in schools and units.* Wiley.
Vygotsky, L. S. (1978). *Mind in society: The development of higher psychological processes.* Harvard University Press.
Willis, P. (1978). *Learning to labour.* Gower.
Wills, D. (1940). Shared responsibility. In D. Wills (Ed.), *Problems of child development* (pp. 411-415). New Education Fellowship.
Wills, D. (1945). *The barns experiment.* Allen and Unwin.
Wills, D. (1960). *Throw away thy rod.* Gollancz.

PART II

Diversity and Inclusion

MICHALIS KAKOS AND PAUL COOPER

3 Identity as Difference: On Distinctiveness, Cool and Inclusion

Introduction

Based on our shared interests in identity, group membership and inclusion and on previous work which explored the appeal of negative affect in adolescents (Cooper & Kakos, 2013), the discussion in this chapter focuses on questions about the significance of difference and individuals' distinctiveness and its relevance to inclusion. The aim of this chapter is to share some of the steps in this jointly developed thinking which led us to a juxtaposition of the interactionist perspectives to identity to those suggested by intersubjective approaches and from there to the exploration of the role of differing in group membership and belonging.

Drawing from our experience in education we reflect on the assumption often embedded in inclusive and especially intercultural education programmes that views diversity in school communities as a challenge which needs to be managed in order for social cohesion to be established or protected (Pagani, 2014). Such view of diversity reflects the understanding of social cohesion as a desirable aim which is associated with the development of generalised trust among members of the group which is known to be negatively impacted by diversity and difference (Hooghe et al., 2009). In the chapter we will suggest that the above views which are largely in agreement with the interactionist approach to identity, effectively promote a model of interculturalism and inclusion which assumes that individuals are in a constant battle with an internalised diversity and in a continuous effort to handle and prioritise multiple identities.

Departing from a problematisation of the interactionist dyadic conceptualisation of individuality based on the distinction between the 'I' and the social selves, we will move to an exploration of the psychoanalytical perspectives in the construction of identity and the process of subjectification. From that angle and reflecting on evidence drawn from short informal discussions with two groups of adolescents, we will initiate a discussion on the prevalence of the concept of distinctiveness and of resistance in subjectification. We will then suggest that the recognition of the significance of distinctiveness may lead our understanding of identity construction much closer to individuals' lived experience, especially in adolescence.

Interactionism: Identity as the Embedment of the 'other' in the Construction of Self

Symbolic interactionism, the theory upon which interactionist approaches are largely based, considers the development of individuals' understanding of social norms and the construction of self and of self-perception as the result of the interaction with others. (see Blumer, 1969; Goffman, 1959; Mead, 1934). Engaged in human interactions, individuals build up 'their perspective lines of conduct by constant interpretation of each other's ongoing lines of action. As participants take account of each other's ongoing acts, they [...] arrest, reorganise, or adjust their own intentions, wishes, feelings, and attitudes; similarly, they [...] judge the fitness of the norms, values, and group prescriptions for the situation being formed by the acts of the others' (Blumer, 1969, p. 66) and evaluate the fitness of their own behaviours to the norms. Interactions, therefore, lead individuals to a process of constant evaluation of behaviours and constant reorganisation of their self-perception and effectively of the 'self' as a social object which arises from the interaction with others (Mead, 1934, pp. 138–140).

At the heart therefore of the process that forms the self is a process of adoption of roles, of performance, of analysing perceptions and expectations, of embedding the 'other' in the construction of the self. Turner describes this as the internalisation of 'self-designations associated with positions that individuals occupy within various social contexts', and this coincides with the identity construction process (Turner, 2013, p. 333). Multiple identities emerge from individuals' involvement in multiple social settings and the corresponding internalisation of 'expectations attached to particular networks of social relationships' (Serpe & Stryker, 2011, p. 232).

In our discussions the above suggestion led us to pose and then to problematise the interactionist responses to two interrelated questions. The first stems from the suggested direct relationship between identities and the interactions within particular social settings. The question concerns the ways that individuals maintain coherence of the self when performing different roles. Interactionism's answer to this question is based on the suggestion about the interplay between the social self and what lies in the core of individuality and referred in symbolic interactionist literature as the 'I' (Blumer, 1969; Mead, 1934). Social actions are in fact initiated by the 'I'. The aim of such actions is to maintain the balance between what lies in the core of individuality and the social self which is prone to the changes resulting from the performance of different identities. The 'I' guides the action of the social self, the action changes the situation and the social self internalises the new situation. The process does not leave the 'I' unaffected but forces it to change through the acting experience. Human agency is located within this process which allows individuals to manipulate their environment and in the interplay between the social self and the 'I' which does not allow individuals to remain unaffected by their own actions. As mentioned above, this interplay is also what secures the sense of continuity in individuals' self-perceptions as they are engaged in the performance of different identities.

The second question is about the cases of role interference (Van Sell et al., 1981) in which 'the pressures of one identity interfere with the performance of another identity' (Settles, 2004, p. 487). For the 'I' to manipulate the situation in a way that leads to the resolution of the conflicts that are caused by role interference there needs to be some hierarchy of identities that guide the action. This hierarchy is based on the evaluation of the importance or psychological attachment that individuals place on their identities and leads to some identities having a more central role in self-perception than others. Research literature attributes a close relationship between this 'role centrality' and individuals' wellbeing (Settles, 2004, p. 487). Structural interactionism, which is a more modern evolution of interactionism, describes the significance that individuals attribute to their identities as identity 'commitment' (Stryker, 1980, 2007). 'Commitment is defined as the degree to which the person's relationships to specified sets of others depends on his or her being a particular kind of person, i.e. occupying a particular position in an organised structure of relationships and playing a particular role. [...] Commitment affects identity salience which in turns affects role-related behavioural choices' (Stryker & Serpe, 1980, p. 207).

From an interactionist perspective therefore the construction of multiple identities is the result of the internalisation of multiple and often conflicting norms, expectations and perspectives, and the handling of these identities is dependent upon the significance that individuals attribute to each of them. Responsible for handling of identities is what lies in the core of individuality, and this exists separately from to the social roles that individuals perform. This core resolves conflicts between identities and guides the social selves to actions which bring changes to the social environment and to themselves. At the root of individual's' socialisation is a process of constant, internalised negotiation of identities and of social roles which represent the norms and the participants' perspectives from and about different social environments, therefore different cultures. Individuality is the host and handler of these identities and cultures, the outcome of multiple conformations and the dialogue between them.

'At the individual level, culture[s] exists in the form of internalised individual-level characteristics' (Chiu et al., 2010, p. 482) stemming from individual's social relations and interculturalism in the internalised dialogue between these cultures. At its best, the project of intercultural education for social inclusion should commence with the support to individuals to develop awareness of their 'individual-level multiculturalism as a tri-dimensional spectrum of the degree to which someone has knowledge of, identification with, and internalization of more than one societal culture' (Vora et al., 2019, p. 500).

From an interactionist perspective, this individual-level multiculturalism can then lead to the development of 'intercultural individuals' who 'exhibit a range of more positive personal attitudes towards diversity' (Kymlicka, 2003, p. 151) through their conscious engagement and handling of their own identity conflicts and of their internalised diversity. Interculturalism, therefore, seen from an interactionist perspective, targets the internalised dialogue between and commitment to identities which aims always to bring balance between the 'I', the multicultural social selves and the social environments with which they interact.

During our discussions which have led to the development of this chapter we followed and then unravelled the interactionist route that leads from the construction to identity to personal interculturalism. Our starting point was a problematisation of the rationale of the significance of the 'Other' to individuality and of the internalisation process, especially as this is perceived by adolescents. By doing so, we integrated in our discussion our doubt about the scope and functionality of the duality that interactionism suggests between the (social) self and the core of individuality (I). Besides, not only in recent literature (see Kögler, 2012) even at the early stages of symbolic interactionism and particularly in Goffman's thought about the 'social self' (1959) there are clear emerging doubts about this duality of 'self' (Bramanan, 1997).

Aborting the Dualism and Doubting about the 'I'

As it has mentioned above, the purpose of the distinction between 'Me' and 'I' is the sense of continuity and coherence that this dualism allows interactionism to explain and the 'running current of awareness' which Mead attributes to the interplay between the two (Mead, 1913). This is of course of major significance since the desire for coherence is essential for survival (see: Guidano & Liotti, 1983; Conway et al., 2004; see also Thomson's case in Sacks, 1986). However, in such case it is worth exploring the sort of understanding that is to be constructed in case that we decide to think outside the confines imposed by the desire for coherence.

We think that such suggestion about the absence of the 'I' brings with it a shift in the role of the Other and arguably elevates the significance of this role. Having lost its 'ground' the concept of self has to be re-defined in reference to the Other and the new concept that seems to be emerging is one that introduces the self as a form of response to the Other. This may not cause problems in understanding the self in the present, but it hinders our understanding of the self as a coherent entity with continuity from the past to the future. The memory of the self could be the link that brings the multiple selves together but the narrative should also depend on an otherness, that which occupies the self at the moment of remembering (Grele, 1985; McMahan, 1986). The state of this constant otherness portrays then a picture of the self which is essentially a negative one: the self exists as a projection of the Other and occupies the void constructed by multiple othernesses. Individuality does not require the solid presence of the interactionist 'I' but exists intersubjectively within the 'larger system created by the mutual interplay between the subjective worlds' (Stolorlow & Atwood, 1996, p. 181). Intersubjectivity suggests that since social behaviours 'invariably take place in relational contexts and should be understood as responses to socially constructed meanings', any attempt to explain 'social behaviours cannot be reduced to individual psychology' (Chiu et al., 2010, p. 483). Indeed, the attention can move away from the individual and focus on the discursive, realised by language concept of the 'subject' (Henriques et al., 1983). In the discursive world which subjects inhibit the self remains in a state of constant subjectivation and otherness and the sense of continuity is not sought in the presence of the 'I' but in the process of subjectivation and in the relationship between the subject and the Other. It is in Butler's suggestions about this relationship that we would like to discuss for the remaining of the theoretical part of this chapter.

For Butler (1993), 'while [..] subjects appear, at least at the level of the everyday or commonsense, to precede their designation, this apparently pre-existing subject is an artefact of its performative constitution' (Youdell, 2006, p. 515). The birth of the subject is located within the process of the disavowal of its dependency to the discourse within which the subject exists, a discourse which 'we never chose but that, paradoxically, initiates and sustains our agency' (Butler, 1997, in Davies, 2006, p. 427). As Davies notes, '... the agentic subject disavows this dependency, [...] because the achievement of autonomy, however illusory it might be, is necessary for the accomplishment of oneself as a recognisable and thus viable subject' (Davies, 2006, p. 427). Davies' observation about the process of disavowal of the subject's dependency brings up the link between autonomy, recognisability and viability of the subject. Indeed, central in Butler's conceptualisation of subjectivation is its contextualisation within a social milieu and the process of recognition of the subject by other subjects (Butler, 1997). It is within this intersubjective context that subjects are recognised and therefore constructed. Such intersubjective understanding of the subject lies very close to Levinas's suggestion: 'For Levinas, our very subjectivity [...] is a function of an existentially prior responsibility: one becomes an "I" by being subject to the other' (Chinnery, 2003, p. 10). A 'dynamic, inter-subjective, constructed moment by moment through social interaction, and, at the same time, subject to existing ideologies and perceived social constraints' (Mayes, 2010, p. 195) understanding of the formation of the subject could integrate the conceptualisation of subjectivation as the subject's birth process and as a discursively constructed confinement of this subject. Unlike individuality, subject can therefore be understood 'not as a known entity, but [...] in process, unfolding or folding up, being done or undone, in relation to the other, again and again' (Davies, 2006, p. 436).

Butler's (1993) suggestion offers an explanation of the subjectivation process and the kind of relationship developed among the subject and the Other (i.e. among subjects). By doing so she offers a description of the void that occupies as the outcome of the resistance of the (existing in discourse) subject to other subjects. This resistance is not the method that leads to autonomy but the reason for the development of the sense of autonomy which, similarly to the subject itself, exists discursively. The subject, therefore, *cannot but resist* and *differ* because it is through this resistance that the subject seeks recognisability and because of which it (intersubjectivity) exists.

Identity, from such intersubjective perspective 'can only occur in an interpersonal context because having an identity is a matter of differentiating oneself from others' (Fowers, 2015, p. 265). Identities are performed as forms of differentiation and recognition and cultures offer the discourses, which contain the scripts, the settings and the roles for such performances. Unlike interactionist approaches, which support a view of interculturalism at individual level as the internalised dialogue and management of identities and of the cultures that they represent, intersubjectivity locates this dialogue in the discursive space of the subjects. While in interactionism the aim of the dialogue is the re-establishment of the balance between the 'I' and the social selves, in intersubjectivity the aim is the differentiation of the subject from other subjects and the recognition. The 'identity commitment' and the resolution of identity conflicts do not need to be based on a premeditated centrality of a particular identity but on the evaluation of the extent to which identities secure recognition. The identity that prevails in such conflicts is not necessarily the one that lead to the re-establishment of a balance but one that offers the greatest recognisability. This is often the identity that is mostly challenged and provokes resistance.

Group Discussions

At this part of this chapter, we will turn our attention to the implications that the suggestion about subjectification and the prevalence of difference might have for identity construction in adolescence, for group culture and intergroup relations. An implication of such suggestion about the central role of difference in the sense of self concerns the understanding of human social behaviour and individuals' affiliations with groups and the sense of 'belonging' which is often at the heart of theories about group membership and identity. We chose to use this sense of 'belonging' and the relationship of individuals with their groups as our entry point in the attempt to build an evidence-based exploration of the role of differing in the ways that young people experience their identities.

Our evidence was collected during short discussions with two groups. The first group was comprised of five sociology students studying the university-entry exams (sixth-form) in a secondary school in North England and the second of four undergraduate students who are members of a University sports club. The discussion with the sixth-form students took place in their school during the lunch break and the discussion with the university students at the university café after a training session. In both cases, our discussions began with an exploration of their affiliation to their groups and the extent and circumstances that this affiliation becomes stronger or weaker. At the second part of the discussions, we outlined our assumption about the significance and role of difference in identity construction and asked for their reflections on the relevance of our assumptions to the ways that they experience their identities.

Belonging as experienced by students in our two groups was clearly dependent on external challenges or comparisons. The members of the sports team described a strong sense of belonging with their group (sports club) which is being heightened during tournaments. The sixth-form students were referring to their identity in contrast to the school pupils and to their distinctiveness in terms of space (their classes occupy the top floor of the school building) and appearance (they are not required to wear school uniforms).

In both groups the discussions led to descriptions of further differentiations. In the case of the sixth form students, participants started describing their distinctiveness to students from other sixth-form courses in the same school, while the university students described sub-groups based on the courses that students attended and their place of origin. In all cases the sub-groups' identities were emerging as a response to questions that were interpreted as attempts to attribute significance of the particular group identity to individuals:

Consistently to the theoretical discussion in this chapter the discussions with the two groups showed the role of recognition in the significance that individuals attribute to identities. Group membership therefore appear to be based less on direct commitment to the group but it seems to be experienced as *affiliations of recognition* that is based on differentiation: Identity is valued when it secures recognition and the corresponding group membership appears as a shared differed to those who are outside of the group (or in other groups). In the words of one of the University students:

- *'I usually wear the [University teams'] uniform when we are out of town. I like it, it's like ... you stand out but you don't seem that you show off or anything because we all wear it'.* [...]
- *Q: Is it important to stand out?*
- *[Laughs]*
- *It is!*
- *You don't want to be like.. to copy anyone* [...]
- *Not too much though.*
- *You want to stand out, but the uniform shows that you stand out for a reason, that you did not try too much. And you are together with others so you all stand out.*

The claim about the importance of *differing* is not new. Brewer (1991, 2003) has developed an evolution-based argumentation that individuals' behaviour and membership in groups responds to two competing human needs: the need of differing and of belonging. Brewer places the basis of her Optimal Distinctiveness Theory (ODT) on the 'premise [...] that the two identity needs (inclusion/assimilation and differentiation/distinctiveness) are independent and work in opposition to motivate group identification' (2003, p. 483). Applied in the analysis of intergroup relationships, ODT has led to suggestions about conditions for groups to achieve the optimal balance between inclusivity and differentiation, avoiding either the detachment of individuals from the group or their assimilation: According to ODT, 'group members will identify most strongly with groups that are neither too differentiated nor too inclusive. That is, the extent to which a group meets either need should also have a curvilinear relation with group identification' (Leonardelli et al., 2010, p. 77).

The theory attributes successful inclusion to the groups' characteristics (more notably size) an suggests that the 'balance between inclusion and differentiation is achieved at the group level, through identification with groups that are both sufficiently inclusive and sufficiently distinct to meet both needs simultaneously' (ibid, p. 67). Groups can either achieve or not the balance in satisfying individual's competing needs while 'the higher the level of inclusiveness at which self-categorisation is made, the more de-personalised the self-concept becomes' (Brewer, 1991, p. 477).

Our discussions with the students did not aim to confirm or reject Brewer's suggestion. However, what we noticed from our discussions is that participants' references to their relationship and affiliation to their groups has little to do with the characteristics of the groups and more to do with the groups from which individuals differentiate: '*I am sixth-from[er] [when I am] in the school canteen* [which is also used by the school pupils] and [I am] a *humanities student when I'm up here [in sixth-form ward]*'. Viewed from such angle, the forces that define inclusion as measured in the level of affiliation of individuals to groups may be predominantly external to the group rather than internal as ODT suggests. Moreover, the dualism that ODT brings forward (competing needs) and the solid point of reference that it suggests in order to explain their function (evolution / human needs) may not be necessary: Differentiation as a key element of subjectification could be considered as the force behind both inclusion and individuality.

Individuals may experience stronger affiliation to certain groups and certain subjects may become dominant in particular stages of individuals' lives. Individuals' response to others' expectations and perceptions that lead to commitment to particular identities may not be based on acceptance as interactionist approaches implies or on the balance between distinctiveness and inclusion as ODT suggests but on a continuous act of resistance and differing which is shared among individuals resisting. Culture, as defined in groups' shared language, sense of humour, history, interpretation of shared experiences can be considered as the outcome of these affiliations of difference and identity may be understood as the affiliation that subjects share since they are produced from the same difference. The dominance of one subject over others and of identities over others depends on the strength of the difference that gives birth to this subject. To follow the course of thought suggested by Butler (1993), the dominance of one identity over others depends on the level of resistance that subjects invest to gain visibility. Or, to describe this differently, we could suggest that the more functional is the difference (in terms of subjects' recognition) the stronger is the subject that is constructed (in terms of dominance over other subjects performed by the same individual). We could therefore suggest that the identity that is resisted (threatened/attacked etc.) is the one that gains in strength and significance for the individuals.

Some Implications

Normal, Abnormal and 'cool'

Distinctiveness and the Need for Uniqueness is a concept which exists in psychology since 1977 (Snyder & Fromkin, 1977) and one which has been applied to a variety of settings including marketing (Pfiffelmann et al., 2023; Ruvio et al., 2008). The conceptualisation of self and the element of difference we think that compliments and explains the need for uniqueness. It can also offer a framework for the understanding of 'cool', an identity-based construct which relies heavily on the balance between distinctiveness (Oyserman, 2009), originality and appeal (Sundar et al., 2014) and is equally significant for consumer research (Sundar et al., 2014) and for studies of adolescence behaviour (Rudolph et al., 2011). Following our analysis, cool can therefore be associated to the behaviour which sits comfortably on the borderline between 'sameness' and 'difference', in a way that is implied in students' quotes about the significance of standing out but 'not too much'. Approaching the concept from an angle that avoids the dichotomy of factors that refer to either desirable or non-desirable attributes (Dar-Nimrod et al., 2012) we suggest that cool incorporates both. If seen as a personality trait (Dar-Nimrod et al., 2012, 2018) cool can describe the distinctiveness that does not alienate individuals from their groups. For this reason, cool does not only change with time (Dar-Nimrod et al., 2012) but it can be experienced differently in different settings even by the same individual. Furthermore, cool may be associated with the appeal and persistence of certain models of behaviour which may be considered as 'dysfunctional' or 'abnormal' (See Cooper & Kakos, 2011, 2013).

Inclusion as Differing

Understanding belonging and group membership as affiliation to common differing, could provide fresh explanation of the effectiveness of particular interventions for inclusive and intercultural education. The effectiveness of Physical Education (PE) with the engagement of students in team sports in intercultural communication which is well evidenced (Carter-Thuillier et al., 2018; Gieß-Stüber, 2010; Grimminger, 2011) but without sufficient recognition of the significance of the role of competition and of shared opposition (Liu & Kramer, 2019). Shifting our attention from the often-unproblematised assumption about the prominence of individuals' need for belonging in explaining participation in groups and intergroup relations to the significance of individuals' constant engagement to resistance and recognition could offer a new perspective and a fresh dynamic to such educational inclusive practices. Such shift can also allow educationalists to recognise processes of exclusion that remain hidden when the inclusivity is sought in the groups' attitudes towards diversity than on the recognition that identification in a given group may grant to its members.

Conclusion

The discussion about identity, is often grounded on the assumption that apart from the social roles performed within such structured or unstructured social groups and beyond the variety of 'senses of similarity' or identities that these assume, there is a solid, autonomous self which guarantees the (sense of) continuity and coherence for the individual. Even in influential theories on identity in adolescence such as that of Erikson (1968) the formation of identity appears as an achievement related to the construction of a solid entity accomplished through a period of psychological moratorium. The failure of achieving this is related to the maintenance of the diversity and flexibility of self-perception described as 'identity diffusion'. Such understanding of identity often justifies the efforts of agents involved with the education of or provision of care to young people to direct them so that they make the 'right identity choices'.

The discussion in this chapter, departing from the problematisation of a core principle of the interactionist approaches to identity construction has raised some questions about the soundness of such understanding of identity. From an intersubjective point of view, the sense of the self as well as the sense of the self's continuity and coherence appear as intersubjective constructions. In the context of such understanding, *difference* and *resistance* appear as being the reasons for the experience of self and *identity* as the projection of self on others who appear to differ similarly. With difference at the heart of self-perception, the choice of identity seems to lead to those perceptions which are associated with recognition of distinctiveness and with resistance. Adolescence does not appear to be a psychosocial moratorium but a factory and a test house of identities and a battleground for the protection of those attracting the most attention. Identity formation in that respect seems not to be the process of 'narrowing down' possible identity choices but the process of identifying the forms of differing which justify such battles.

The analysis in this part is based on limited evidence collected almost opportunistically. Our ambition has been to support the problematisation of the traditional approaches to identity and the assumptions that are often dominant in the conceptual frameworks of inclusive and intercultural education programmes. Further research is necessary to examine the intersubjective lived experiences of young people with regards to the development and performance of their identities based on appropriate (broadly ethnographic) methodologies that allow 'lived intercultural experiences of all involved parties to emerge' (Holliday & MacDonald, 2020, p. 635).

References

Blumer, H. (1969). *Symbolic interactionism: Perspective and method*. Berkley: University of California Press.
Branaman, A. (1997). Goffman's social theory. In C. Lemert & A. Branaman (Eds), *The Goffman reader* (pp. xiv–ixxxii). Blackwell.

Brewer, M. (1991). The social self: On being the same and different at the same time. *Personality and Social Psychology Bulletin*, *17*(5), 475–482.
Brewer, M. (2003). Optimal distinctiveness, social identity and the self. In M. R. Leary & J. P. Tangney (Eds), Handbook of self and identity (pp. 480–491). The Guilford Press.
Butler, J. (1993). *Bodies that matter: On the discursive limits of 'sex'*. Routledge.
Butler, J. (1997). *The psychic life of power: Theories in subjection*. Stanford University Press.
Carter-Thuillier, B., López-Pastor, V., Gallardo-Fuentes, F., & Carter-Beltran, J. (2018). Immigration and social inclusion: Possibilities from school and sports. In T. N. Sequeira (Ed.), *Immigration and development* (pp. 57–74). IntechOpen.
Chinnery, A. (2003). Aesthetics of surrender: Levinas and the disruption of agency in moral education. *Studies in Philosophy and Education*, *22*(1), 5–17.
Chiu, C.-Y., Gelfand, M. J., Yamagishi, T., Shteynberg, G., & Wan, C. (2010). Intersubjective culture: The role of intersubjective perceptions in cross-cultural research. *Perspectives on Psychological Science*, *5*(4), 482–493. <https://doi.org/10.1177/1745691610375562>.
Conway, M. A., Singer, J. A., & Tagini, A. (2004). The self and autobiographical memory: Correspondence and coherence. *Social Cognition*, *22*(5), 495–537.
Cooper, P., & Kakos, M. (2011). *Is it sometimes cool to appear to be depressed? Identity and negative affect among adolescents*. Paper presented in ECER, Freie Universität Berlin, 13–16 September 2011.
Cooper, P., & Kakos, M. (2013). 'Man you've been a naughty boy, you let your face grow long': On the celebration of negative affect in adolescence. *International Journal of Emotional Education*, *5*(1), 3–16.
Dar-Nimrod, I., Ganesan, A., & MacCann, C. (2018). Coolness as a trait and its relations to the Big Five, self-esteem, social desirability and action orientation. *Personality and Individual Differences*, *121*, 1–6. <https://doi.org/10.1016/j.paid.2017.09.012>.
Dar-Nimrod, I., Hansen, I. G., Proulx, T., Lehman, D. R., Chapman, B. P., & Duberstein, P. R. (2012). Coolness: An empirical investigation. *Journal of Individual Differences*, *33*(3), 175–185. <http://dx.doi.org/10.1027/1614-0001/a000088>.
Davies, B. (2006). Subjectification: The relevance of Butler's analysis for education. *British Journal of Sociology of Education*, *27*(4), 425–438.
Erikson, E. (1968). *Identity: Youth and crisis*. Norton.
Fowers, B. J. (2015). Intersubjectivity and identity. In B. J. Fowers (Ed.), *The evolution of ethics: Palgrave studies in the theory and history of psychology* (pp. 95–130). Palgrave Macmillan. <https://doi.org/10.1057/9781137344663_5>.

Gieß-Stüber, P. (2010). Development of intercultural skills through sport and physical education in Europe. In W. Gasparini & A. Cometti (Eds), *Sport facing the test of cultural diversity: Integration and intercultural dialogue in Europe: Analysis and practical examples* (pp. 23–29). Council of Europe.

Goffman, E. (1959, reprint 1990). *The presentation of self in everyday life.* Penguin Books.

Grele, R. (1979). Listen to their voices: Two case studies in the interpretation of oral history interviews. *Oral History, 7*(1), 33–43.

Grimminger, E. (2011). Intercultural competence among sports and PE teachers: Theoretical foundations and empirical verification. *European Journal of Teacher Education, 34*(3), 317–337. <https://doi.org/10.1080/02619768.2010.546834>.

Guidano, V. F., & Liotti, G. (1983). *Cognitive processes and emotional disorders: A structural approach to psychotherapy.* Guilford Press.

Henriques, J., Hollway, W., Urwin, C., Venn, C., & Walkerdine, V. (1998). *Changing the subject: Psychology, social regulation and subjectivity* (2nd edn). Routledge.

Holliday, A., & MacDonald, M. (2020). Researching the intercultural: Intersubjectivity and the problem with postpositivism. *Applied Linguistics, 4*(5), 621–639.

Hooghe, M., Reeskens, T., Stolle, D., & Trappers, A. (2009). Ethnic diversity and generalized trust in Europe: A cross-national multilevel study. *Comparative Political Studies, 42*(2), 198–223. <https://doi.org/10.1177/0010414008325286>.

Kögler, H.-H. (2012). Agency and the other: On the intersubjective roots of self-identity. *New Ideas in Psychology, 30*(1), 47–64. <https://doi.org/10.1016/j.newideapsych.2010.03.010>.

Kymlicka, W. (2003). Multicultural states and intercultural citizens. *Theory and Research in Education, 1*(2), 147–169.

Leonardelli, G. J., Pickett, C. L., & Brewer, M. B. (2010). Optimal distinctiveness theory: A framework for social identity, social cognition, and intergroup relations. *Advances in Experimental Social Psychology, 43*, 63–113.

Liu, Y., & Kramer, E. (2019). Conceptualizing the other in intercultural encounters: Review, formulation, and typology of the other-identity. *Howard Journal of Communications, 30*(5), 446–463. <https://doi.org/10.1080/10646175.2018.1532850>.

Mayes, P. (2010). The discursive construction of identity and power in the critical classroom: Implications for applied critical theories. *Discourse & Society, 21*(2), 189–210. <https://doi.org/10.1177/0957926509353846>

McMahan, E. (1986). *Elite oral history discourse: A study of cooperation and coherence.* University of Alabama Press.

Mead, G. H. (1913). The social self. *Journal of Philosophy, Psychology and Scientific Methods, 10*, 374–380.

Mead, G. H. (1934). *Mind, self and society.* University of Chicago Press.
Oyserman, D. (2009). Identity-based motivation and consumer behaviour. *Journal of Cosnumer Psychology, 19*, 276–279. <https://doi.org/10.1016/j.jcps.2009.06.001>.
Pagani, C. (2014). Diversity and social cohesion. *Intercultural Education, 25*(4), 300–311. <http://dx.doi.org/10.1080/14675986.2014.926158>.
Pfiffelmann, J., Pfeuffer, A., Dens, N., & Soulez, S. (2023). Unique ... like everyone else: Effects and mechanisms of personalization appeals in recruitment advertising. *International Journal of Advertising.* <http://dx.doi.org/10.1080/02650487.2023.2203577>.
Qualifications and Curriculum Authority (QCA). (1998). *Education for citizenship and the teaching of democracy in schools.* Qualifications and Curriculum Authority.
Rudolph, K. D., Abaied, J. L., Flynn, M., Sugimura, N., & Agoston, A. M. (2011). Developing relationships, being cool, and not looking like a loser: Social goal orientation predicts children's response to peer aggression. *Child Development, 82*(5), 1518–1530. <https://doi.org/10.1111/j.1467-8624.2011.01631.x>.
Ruvio, A., Shoham, A., & Brenčič, M. (2008). Consumers' need for uniqueness: Short-form scale development and cross-cultural validation. *International Marketing Review, 25*(1), 33–53. <http://dx.doi.org/10.1108/02651330810851872>.
Sacks, O. (1986). *The man who mistook his wife for a hat, and other clinical tales.* Picador.
Serpe, R. T., & Stryker, S. (2011). The symbolic interactionist perspective and identity theory. In S. J. Schwartz, K. Luyckx, & V. L. Vignoles (Eds), *Handbook of identity theory and research* (pp. 225–248). Springer. <https://doi.org/10.1007/978-1-4419-7988-9_10>.
Snyder, C. R., & Fromkin, H. L. (1977). Abnormality as a positive characteristic: The development and validation of a scale measuring need for uniqueness. *Journal of Abnormal Psychology, 86*(5), 518–527.
Stolorow, R. D., & Atwood, G. E. (1996). The intersubjective perspective. *Psychoanalytic Review, 83*, 181–194.
Stryker, S. (2007). Identity theory and personality theory: Mutual relevance. *Journal of Personality, 75*, 1083–1102.
Stryker, S., & Serpe, R. T. (1982). Commitment, identity salience, and role behavior: Theory and research example. In W. Ickes & E. S. Knowles (Eds), *Personality, roles, and social behavior* (pp. 199–218). New York, NY: Springer.
Turner, J. (2013). *Contemporary sociological theory.* Sage.
Van Sell, M., Brief, A. P., & Schuler, R. S. (1981). Role conflict and role ambiguity: Integration of the literature and directions for future research. *Human Relations, 34*, 43–71.

Vora, D., Martin, L., Fitzsimmons, S. R., Pekerti, A. A., Lakshman, C., & Raheem, S. (2019). Multiculturalism within individuals: A review, critique, and agenda for future research. *Journal of International Business Studies, 50,* 499–524. <https://doi.org/10.1057/s41267-018-0191-3>.

Youdell, D. (2006). Subjectivation and performative politics – Butler thinking Althusser and Foucault: Intelligibility, agency and the raced-nationed-religioned subject of education. *British Journal of Sociology of Education, 27*(4), 511–528.

BRAHM NORWICH

4 The Biopsychosocial Model and What It Means for Understanding Inclusion in Education

Introduction

This chapter focuses on two specific pieces of Paul Cooper's writing from nineteen and fifteen years ago respectively, namely his ideas about the biopsychosocial model and how he developed and used this perspective in unique ways to expand our thinking about inclusion and inclusive education. This will provide the opportunity to show the detail of his analyses and way he engaged in the key debates going on in the field. It will also illustrate the continuing relevance of the arguments Paul voiced to current issues and concerns. Paul's intellectual approach has been to oppose what he sees as false oppositions or dichotomies and this is something I have learned from and shared with him. The biopsychosocial model was for him a way to combine and bring together a more complex synthesis not just as an intellectual exercise, but as critical to enhancing educational practice, especially for those with disability and difficulties.

A Critical Discussion of Education, ADHD and the Biopsychosocial (BPS) Perspective

Paul Cooper's paper on the biopsychosocial perspective (Cooper, 2008) focuses on ADHD to propose a BPS model or what is called here a 'paradigm' as a way forward to address controversies amongst educationalists. Its argument had and continues to have much wider significance for the field of special educational needs and inclusive education. The main point in the paper was to show how the polarity between biological and social explanations for learning and behaviour problems had become redundant and unhelpful. ADHD it was stated was influenced by both biology and the social environment and indeed was 'socially constructed'. But, this notion of social construction was not like the one adopted by the social model advocates referenced in the paper and still widely used in the 2020s. Shakespeare (2018, p. 68), for example, refers to the social model of disability as 'the idea that people are disabled by society, rather than by their bodies'. What motivated Paul was the negativity towards the ADHD concept based on what he saw as 'outdated thinking and a lack of understanding of the diagnosis and the biopsychosocial paradigm through which it can be usefully understood' (p. 457).

Before examining the arguments about a social or a BPS model of ADHD, it worth exploring the usage of the terms in these models in written publications generally and in relation to academic research publications in education. Using the google ngram viewer system shows that the phrase 'social model of disability' is used 114 times more in those texts covered within the google system than the phrase 'biopsychosocial model of disability' published in 2019. In addition, references to the phrase 'social model of disability; increased 2.6 times from 2000 to 2019. By contrast, the use of the phrase 'biopsychosocial model of disability' increased more rapidly by 9.3 times, over the same period. Though this analysis is confined to those ngram accessed books in English, it does show that the 'social model' was used in this corpus considerably more than the 'BPS model'. This is so even when the 'BPS model' had a greater increase in usage compared to the 'social model' over this almost two-decade period. This picture is repeated when examining research literature references in education using the Education Research Complete database (ERC). In a search for literature with the terms 'inclusive education or inclusion or mainstreaming or integration' and either 'biopsychosocial model' or 'social model', it was found that there were thirteen times as many references for social model than BPS model.

It is clear from these analyses that Paul Cooper's position has not been widely adopted since the 2000s and into the late 2010s, despite the international interest in the WHO International Classification of Functioning (ICF), which adopts a BPS model of disability (Hollenweger, 2012). My argument here is that this does not detract from the value and importance of the arguments in his paper. I am not going into the details of the case for the usefulness and risks in the use of medical classification systems that include ADHD as the most prevalent of childhood behaviour disorders. Cooper's 2008 paper does this, and no doubt since then the current state of knowledge about ADHD has changed. What I will focus on is the argument made by Paul Cooper about the involvement of biological processes in functioning that comes to be identified as ADHD. Here he considered evidence for there being a problem in the response inhibition system, involving neuropsychological executive functioning mechanisms implicating physiological processes in the frontal lobes of the brain. In addition, he also implicates the genetic studies that have shown a much greater incidence of ADHD among identical than non-identical twins and among children who are biologically related as opposed to adopted. What he resists is the polarising between recognising these biological processes on human behaviour and the social processes; the *either – or* in favour of the *both – and* perspective. This is a central point in the commentary I am making of Paul Cooper's positions and one which will be made too in relation to his ideas about inclusion in education below. The BPS model he is advocating rejects a biological determinism and represents biological factors as being mediated by psychosocial processes; the biological is subjected to social construction at various social and psychological levels. See Figure 4.1 which represents this kind of BPS model. In this respect the BPS model he advocates has strong links to Bronfenbrenner's bioecological model (Bronfenbrenner & Morris, 2006). It is notable that many references to Bronfenbrenner's ecological model have tended to also split the biological from the psycho-social (Tudge et al., 2009).

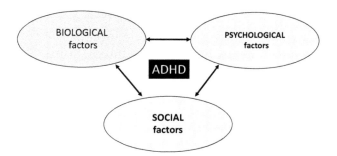

Figure 4.1. Factors in interaction in the bio-psycho-social model of ADHD

Critical reactions to ADHD have involved the dismissal of ADHD by some as a medical construct that individualises educational failure and disruptive behaviour. Part of the aversion to ADHD has been its use to legitimise the practice of using drugs as a form of social control of defiant children. Some argued this approach represented wrong-headed pseudo-science. The argument which Paul Cooper focussed on was the assertion that this individualised these problems, distract from how schools and teachers were involved in these problems, and so absolve them of responsibility to provide relevant opportunities for these groups. He countered this argument by claiming that the BPS model recognises that schools are a major setting through which institutional control and pedagogical practices contribute to the construction of ADHD. In his argument for a more complex BPS model, he countered the arguments of authors like Slee (1995) who were critical of what they portrayed as 'The monism of locating the nature of [classroom] disruption in the neurological infrastructure of the child is myopic and convenient' (Slee, 1995, p. 74).

Slee has continued this critical line of argument with his more recent views about the language of special educational needs in referring to 'the saturation of our discourse and thinking with the quasi-medical posturing of special educational needs. The conceptual foundations and usage of terms like special educational needs passes without a second thought' (Slee, 2018; p. 78).

Paul Cooper's thorough response to four challenges from the critical perspective continue to be very relevant to the current circumstances.

Firstly, it has been claimed that the ADHD diagnosis is somehow bogus or 'illicit' because there is an absence of neuro-scientific evidence. In this article he illustrates how this is 'patently untrue' (p. 463). Secondly, ADHD is sometimes claimed to be an example of biological determinism, a claim which expresses a fear of determinism and its associated denial of human agency. Here he has sympathy with this fear but shows how this is not well founded as regards developmental opportunities, given the interaction between biological inheritance and environmental factors in the development of behavioural difficulties.

Paul Cooper argued that not only were there several biological pathways implicated in the development of ADHD, but that ADHD is not biologically determined in the simplistic sense suggested by some; see the Slee quote above. He turns the argument by ADHD critics about ADHD diverting attention from school factors against their position. He suggests that portraying ADHD as an example of biological determinism, itself diverts attention from converting a biopsychosocial account of ADHD into pedagogical and other interventions. By knowing more about the biological, psychological and social factors in ADHD enables us, he argued, to avoid aggravating experienced difficulties and promoting educational engagement.

The third challenge he addressed was that an ADHD 'diagnosis' rests on value-laden, culturally-specific judgements about behavioural or cognitive norms. Here Paul Cooper adopts a perspective, not often found in debates about behaviour difficulties and school education norms. He recognised that children who are biologically predisposed to develop ADHD can be at a disadvantage by culturally based assumptions about appropriate school and classroom behaviour. But, this, he argues, does not reflect on the clinicians who identify ADHD, but reflects on the weaknesses of, what he called, 'Western mass education'. This issue is about whether to change the educational environment to accommodate the student or to change the student to enable him or her to engage with an unchanging environment.

As Paul Cooper recognised the attempt is often made to combine environmental and individual changes. He suggested that using medication can be seen as the failure of the school to make changes that enable the student with ADHD to engage effectively. The implications for those wanting to make schools more inclusive is to learn the lesson that ADHD teaches about shaping the educational environment to improve learning opportunities. In discussing how he approached this challenge, it is also notable that some psychologists have adopted more recently a BPS model of ADHD and supplemented the social aspects with a focus on the cultural aspects that relate to the mental health needs of culturally and linguistically diverse children and young people (Pham, 2015).

The fourth challenge Paul Cooper responded to was that accepting an ADHD diagnosis 'legitimise[s] the practice of drugging defiant children into docility' (Skidmore, 2004, p. 4). To this he points out that informed opinion does not consider medication for ADHD as an essential treatment, and that whatever is decided is to be in the context of a multimodal treatment programme that includes psychosocial and educational interventions. In his paper he refers to the UK guidance from 2000 and this is still the current guidelines (NICE, 2018). How parents participate in intervention selection is also illustrated in Pham (2015). The linked and final challenge he dealt with was that ADHD represents the wrongful medicalisation of defiance in school children. Here Paul Cooper questioned the link between defiance and the functional issues associated with ADHD. He suggested that defiance is better considered as a cognitive distortion affecting social engagement rather than a deficit in executive functioning associated with ADHD. So, not complying with parent wishes is seen as non-volitional and not to be confused with defiance. For him what was concerning was the 'high moral tone' (Pham, 2015, p. 470) which concealed limited understanding about ADHD that he believed could be dangerous.

A Crucial Difference between the Social and BPS Models

In defending the BPS model from critical arguments, Paul Cooper did not examine the ideological or value basis for the knowledge claims in these debates. From a critical perspective, it has been suggested by

Slee and Weiner (2001) that it is possible to identify two groups of researchers, which they characterise in these terms, namely those who work within, what they call the 'positivist paradigm', accept the way things are, attempt to make marginal reforms and who criticise 'full inclusion' as ideological; and those who see inclusive education as cultural politics and call for educational reconstruction. This distinction between a positivist/technical versus cultural political position can be aligned with one between an investigatory versus an emancipatory perspective to research about disability (Oliver, 1999). Oliver frames the research-as-investigation as the dominant form of social research which is unacceptable to oppressed groups, such as those with disabilities, who aim to collectively empower themselves. In this perspective the social model of disability expresses the emancipatory stance which is pursued through cultural politics. This contrasts with a technical – interventionist perspective that derives from what Slee and Weiner (2001) call a 'positivist paradigm' and is associated with what is called a medical or a biomedical model. It can be seen that this dichotomy between research stances embraces the splitting which Paul Cooper argued against.

Figure 4.2 below represents these distinct research stances as adopting emancipatory or investigatory values, while showing their focus and linked assumptions. With emancipatory values the focus is on reducing the oppression of the vulnerable with this being done through collective socio-political action and in doing so entailing a causal assumption that it is the dominant social system that oppresses. With investigatory values, the main focus is on identifying complex causal models of a phenomenon and in doing so assumes that this knowledge can be used for subsequent improvement interventions.

One of the main arguments in this chapter is that there are links and common elements to these two basic value positions, so raising questions about the split and opposition between them. Both connect knowledge with action for social change, on one hand, and both assume some causal processes, on the other. The difference is in the assumptions of their focus. Identifying complex causal processes (e.g. that includes social processes as part of a BPS perspective) is the primary focus of the investigatory stance, while change depends on applying this knowledge in interventions. This stance represents an outsider-spectator-intervenor perspective. By contrast, reducing the oppression of the vulnerable is the primary focus of the emancipatory stance, with this being through collective political and social action. This stance represents an insider-participator perspective. So, while distinct, there are connections to be recognised between them which can help to understand what the social stands for in these two models. The social in the social model stands for where change is to be focussed: in the socio-political arena. The social, by contrast, in the BPS model stands for the social factors that need to be understood in their interaction with bio-psychological causal factors.

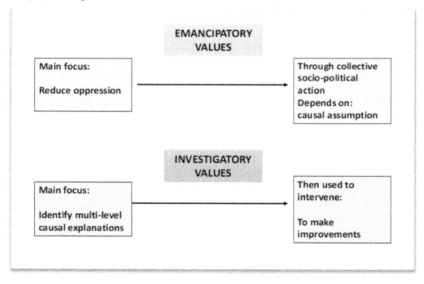

Figure 4.2. Value bases underlying different research stances

Making use of the distinction between insider-outsider role perspectives enables us to see how these different value stances can be connected and not seen as opposites to select between. As Paul Cooper argued in his 2008 paper, informed opinion does not consider medication for ADHD as an essential treatment/intervention; the BPS model implies multi-modal methods including psychosocial and educational interventions (NICE, 2018). Intervention/treatment acceptability is also an important consideration when considering individual children with identified ADHD from a BPS perspective, as illustrated in Pham's (2015) case study. This implies that parents and young people will participate in action decisions, which gives them an insider role. However, the social model goes beyond insider participation at the individual level, involving also collective participation at institutional and societal levels. This is where the BPS model could be open to insider participation beyond the individual level, that is, to see the value of institutional and societal participation as well. And, as the BPS can be open to the collective action of the social model, so the social model can be open to the outsider perspective's recognition of multilevel causal processes (including the bio-psychological levels) and their associated interventions.

Inclusion as a Buzzword

In this 2008 paper Paul Cooper suggested that the use of insights from the BPS model in developing educational provision is likely to lead to a more genuinely inclusive education system. This was written after an earlier editorial he wrote in the journal *Emotional and Behavioural Difficulties* in 2004 (Cooper, 2004a). Here he pointed to the overuse and misuse of the word inclusion, suggesting that it will lose its meaning and that the purposes for which it was coined will become neglected. One way of challenging this misuse, he mentioned, was to be vigilant about how it is used and to call for greater clarity. In this editorial he stated that social inclusion is about active participation and engagement with other people. With inclusive education, he continued, it is not just about social inclusion, but an individual's active engagement in formal learning processes. Here Paul Cooper goes beyond common ideas about inclusion which are defined in terms of social and academic participation (as in the Inclusion Index; Booth & Ainscow, 2011), by clarifying that it is also about academic and social engagement. From this it was clear that inclusion was more than both location/placement and social interaction with other people; it was also about personal engagement with others and with formal learning.

Paul Cooper was not alone in linking engagement with inclusion, he shared this with Mary Warnock, the chair of the Warnock Committee which in 1978 set out new policies about the education of children and young people with disabilities and difficulties (Warnock, 2005). In her 2005 policy paper she rejected the idea of educational inclusion as about 'all children under the same roof'. She preferred a learning concept of inclusion, which was about: 'including all children in the common educational enterprise of learning, wherever they learn best' (Warnock, 2005). Though she does not use the term 'engagement' as such, her notion of *learning where done best* connects with 'engagement' and prioritises this over placement, a view which was also adopted later by Paul for the area of education of children and young people with social, emotional and behaviour difficulties (Cooper & Jacobs, 2011).

Paul Cooper drew on the psychological ideas of Marjorie Boxall in the Boxall Profile (Bennathan & Boxall, 2003) to connect Inclusion with engagement, as he mentioned in his 2004 editorial. For him engagement was at the heart of educational inclusion from a cognitive perspective. He adopted the five subskills of what the Boxall Profile termed 'the organization of experience': whether the child gives purposeful attention, participates constructively, connects up experiences, shows insightful involvement and engages cognitively with peers. Within this framework he recognised that children with social, emotional and behavioural difficulties (SEBD) can have problems with some or all of these skills. So, it can be argued that the child who experiences SEBD is socially, emotionally and cognitively excluded from what is going in class lessons; with SEBD being framed as a barrier to inclusion. This concept of a barrier is very different to that proposed from a social model perspective as in the Inclusion Index (Booth & Ainscow, 2011), in which barriers are only external to the person. But, Paul Cooper does not draw the conclusion that children with SEBD can never be 'included'. Here he makes the distinction between inclusion-as-location and inclusion-as-engagement, with the implication that in some cases when there is not mainstream class inclusion this does not mean there cannot be some engagement inclusion. He also reminded us that inclusion is such that nobody is ever fully included in any situation all the time. In this sense his ideas resemble Qvortrup and Qvortrup's (2018) argument that inclusion and exclusion are connected through peoples' simultaneous involvement in different social arenas. With social interactions involving negotiations in all situations, Paul Cooper argued that any episode can result in tensions and the rejection of the people involved. This is a feature of our lives and in this respect the child experiencing SEBD is no different from others. However, he pointed out that the child or young person with a SEBD is at greater risk of rejection or exclusion, which may be attributed to individual characteristics in interaction with social circumstances (in line with a BPS model).

Using this notion of engagement, he also approached the questions of teaching children and young people with SEBD in terms of the BPS model. In avoiding a focus just on problems located in the student, he adopted an interactionist perspective that combined specialist teaching knowledge about individual differences with teachers' practical thinking about decision-making that led to adapted teaching (Cooper, 2004b). He reviewed in this 2004 chapter and in his later 2008 paper discussed above, the various teaching strategies that research had shown to promote further engagement for children with ADHD. It is useful here to compare his engagement perspective to a well-known 'Inclusive Pedagogy (IP) framework for participation in classrooms' developed by Florian and Black-Hawkins (2011). This framework in covering access, collaboration, achievement and diversity aimed to extend what was typically available in the classroom community to all. It avoided having learning activities for most being alongside different activities for some who experience difficulties. It also proposed differentiation by pupil choice for everyone while rejecting ability grouping. This is an approach that required flexibility to be driven by need and not curriculum coverage, while seeing difficulties in learning as professional challenges rather than learner deficits.

Though Paul Cooper's perspective agreed with some elements of this inclusive pedagogy framework (e.g. flexibility and responding to learning difficulties as a challenge), his does not accept the *either-or* polarity at the core of the framework with the adoption of only one option: differentiation by choice v. by grouping and only opting for the former, or seeing learning difficulties as a professional challenge v. learner deficits and opting only for the challenge option). This IP framework reflects the medical v social model polarity that he argued against while favouring a BPS model. Based on his approach of seeing social and academic engagement as being at the heart of educational and social inclusion, he believed that it followed that: 'students are best placed in educational settings where they have access to and support for maximum social and academic engagement'. (Cooper, 2004, p. 222). In his view, this meant that there was no simple way to decide about the provision setting. For some pupils this meant access to various forms of provision, but always a detailed analysis of individual capabilities and needs as well as what provision affords should determine the decisions.

Conclusion

This chapter has focussed on two of Paul Cooper's papers in which he explained and justified his ideas about the biopsychosocial model and how he developed and used this perspective in unique ways to expand our thinking about inclusion and inclusive education. Through relating and contrasting these with other contemporary and current ideas I hope to have shown his distinctive and insightful contribution. I have also tried to extend his adoption of a *both-and* rather than an *either-or* approach by discussing the epistemological and value bases of different models, on one hand, and how difference and distinction does not imply irreconcilable opposition between the key models in the field.

References

Bennathan, M., & Boxall, M. (2003). *The Boxall profile.* SEBDA.
Booth, T., & Ainscow, M. (2011). *Index for inclusion: Developing learning and participation in schools* (3rd edn). CSIE.

Bronfenbrenner, U., & Morris, P. (2006). The bioecological model of human development. In W. Damon & R. M. Lerner (Eds), *Handbook of child psychology: Vol. 1. Theoretical models of human development* (6th edn, pp. 793–828). Wiley.

Cooper, P. (2004a). Is 'inclusion' just a buzz-word?. *Emotional and Behavioural Difficulties, 9*(4), 219–222. <https://doi.org/10.1177/1363275204051391>.

Cooper, P. (2004b). AD/HD. In A. Lewis & B. Norwich (Eds), *Special teaching for special children? Pedagogies for inclusion* (pp. 121–137). Open University Press.

Cooper, P. (2008). Like alligators bobbing for poodles? A critical discussion of education, ADHD and the biopsychosocial perspective. *Journal of Philosophy of Education, 42*(3–4), 457–474.

Cooper, P., & Jacobs, B. (2011). *From inclusion to engagement: Helping students engage with schooling through policy and practice*. Wiley.

Florian, L., & Black-Hawkins, K. (2011). Exploring inclusive pedagogy. *British Educational Research Journal, 37*(5), 813–828.

Hollenweger, J. (2012). Using the international classification of functioning, disability and health children and youth version in education systems. *American Journal of Physical Medicine and Rehabilitation, 91*(13), 97–102.

NICE. (2018). *Attention deficit hyperactivity disorder: Diagnosis and management NICE guidelines*. Published: 14 March 2018. Retrieved from <www.nice.org.uk/guidance/ng87>

Oliver, M. (1999). Final accounts and the parasite people. In M. Corker & S. French (Eds), *Disability discourse*. Open University Press.

Pham, A. V. (2015). Understanding ADHD from a biopsychosocial-cultural framework: A case study. *Contemporary School Psychology, 19*, 54–62.

Qvortrup, A., & Qvortrup, L. (2018). Inclusion: Dimensions of inclusion in education. *International Journal of Inclusive Education, 22*(7), 803–817.

Shakespeare, T. (2018). *Disability: The basics*. Routledge.

Skidmore, D. (2004). *Inclusion*. Open University Press.

Slee, R. (1995). *Changing theories and practices of discipline*. Falmer.

Slee, R. (2018). *Inclusive education isn't dead, it just smells funny*. Routledge.

Slee, R., & Weiner, G. (2001). Education reform and reconstruction as a challenge to research genres: Reconsidering school effectiveness research and inclusive schooling. *School Effectiveness and School Improvement, 12*(1), 83–98. <https://doi.org/10.1076/sesi.12.1.83.3463>.

Tudge, J. R. H., Mokrova, I., Hatfield, B. E., & Karnik, R. B. (2009). Uses and misuses of Bronfenbrenner's bioecological theory of human development. *Journal of Family Theory & Review, 1*, 198–210.

Warnock, M. (2005). *Special educational needs: A new look*. Philosophy of education society of Great Britain, impact series no. 11.

PAUL DOWNES

5 Reframing Cooper's Emotional-Relational, Commodification and Biopsychosocial Concerns as a Spatial Turn towards Concentric Systems of Inclusion

Introduction

A range of strands in Paul Cooper's interdisciplinary work across psychology, education and philosophy explore key themes of what can be construed as an emotional-relational turn for education (Downes, 2011). This emotional-relational turn invites an acceleration of focus on the need for system reform regarding shift towards supportive rather than authoritarian relationships in schools and a concern with social and emotional education (SEE), including nurture rooms. A pervasive feature of these concerns is with removing a climate of fear in education, whether for students (Cefai & Cooper, 2010) or also teachers, regarding their agency for curricular implementation in an English context (Cooper, 2008a). Agency is another frequent theme in Cooper's work, not only regarding students' and teachers' voices. It also underpins his concerns with commodification in education, as well as with the need to go beyond genetic or environmental determinism, as part of a biopsychosocial model for developmental and educational psychology.

This chapter will argue that these currents in Cooper's cross-disciplinary thought can be reframed in specific spatial systems terms, as part of a critical spatial hermeneutics to promote agency and inclusion in education. In doing so, this is resonant with a spatial turn for education investigating connective potentials in space through 'new spaces of engagement wherein adult–child relations get reconfigured' (Mannion, 2007, p. 410). As part of a proposed spatial turn for education, Ferrare and Apple (2010, p. 216) seek understandings of 'spatial processes in education [;] we not only need these "new" theories, but we also need to employ methodological tools that "think" spatially'. The proposed critical spatial hermeneutics in this article offers a particular scrutiny of inclusion in education as a spatial concept, as well as *systems* as being spatial (Downes, 2020a).

This interrogation of relational spaces in education occurs with regard to concrete cross-cultural structures of diametric and concentric space (Downes, 2009, 2013, 2020a), building on Lévi-Strauss' structural anthropology. A conception of space as active and patterned, through concentric and diametric structures, challenges Descartes' treatment of space, so influential in the history of Western thought. He referred to 'empty space, which almost everyone is convinced is mere nonentity' (Descartes, 1954, p. 200). Recognition of concentric and diametric spatial systems does not treat space as empty and homogenous.

To some degree, space is already explicitly embraced in central themes of Cooper's work. This is done, most obviously, through his reviews on nurture rooms in schools (Cefai & Cooper, 2011; Cooper et al., 2001), a thoroughly spatial concern with safe spaces in school settings to nurture children's individual differences, emotional and social development. Another abiding preoccupation in Cooper's work is that with inclusion. He advocates for an inclusive school culture 'based on a commitment to valuing all pupils as members of the school community ... to ensure all pupils have access to the experience of success' (Cooper, 2008a, p. 17). It is to be highlighted that inclusion and exclusion are spatial concepts (Downes, 2020a), as well as being linked to economic issues of poverty. Likewise, marginalisation is also a spatial concept, as Massey (2005) foregrounds; marginalisation assumes distance and exclusion in her recognition that space is broader than simply a focus on place. A further example of spatially imbued thinking in Cooper's work is his account of curricular reforms in England through the spatial metaphor of 'a straitjacket' (2008, p. 16), imposed upon teachers, to thwart their agency and capacity to interpret the curriculum. Yet all of these thematic concerns with agency, removal of fear and with space can go further, as part of a critical spatial hermeneutic to interrogate expanded horizons related to Cooper's work.

A Cross-Cultural Framework of Contrasting Concentric and Diametric Spatial Systems

A critical spatial systems framework builds on the cross-cultural observations of spatial structures of diametric and concentric spaces, highlighted by Lévi-Strauss (1963, 1973). A diametric spatial structure is one where a circle is split in half by a line which is its diameter or where a square or rectangle is similarly divided into two equal halves (see Figure 5.1). In a concentric spatial structure, one circle is inscribed in another larger circle (or square); in pure form, the circles share a common central point (see Figure 5.2).

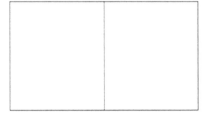

Figure 5.1. Diametric dualism

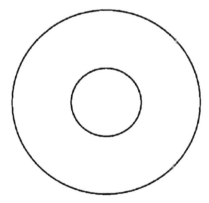

Figure 5.2. Concentric dualism

Lévi-Strauss (1963) cites a range of examples of the concentric spatial opposition observed by different anthropologists. These include: the village plan of Omarakana in the Trobriand Islands, published by Malinowski; the Baduj of western Java and the Negri-Sembilan of the Malay peninsula, observed by de Jong; the village of the Winnebago tribe observed by Radin. Jung (1936/1985) locates the concentric mandala structure in Buddhist, Hindu and Christian traditions. Concentric structures can be found also in the well-known Chinese yin/yang symbol, as well as in Celtic, African, Japanese, Russian, Scandinavian, ancient Greek and Estonian contexts, including Jewish and Islamic traditions (Downes 2012, 2020a). The contrasting structural relation of diametric spatial opposition has also been observed cross-culturally, by Lévi-Strauss (1962); he notes that examples of diametric dualism 'abound' (Lévi-Strauss, 1962, p. 135), citing specific tribes in North and South America. Moreover, the simple 'subjective' (Leach, 1965/2000, p. 111) everyday cross-cultural oppositions between 'good' and 'bad' are structured in a diametric oppositional way.

A purportedly key distinguishing feature of concentric and diametric spaces, observed by Lévi-Strauss (1973), is that they tend to coexist in 'functional relation' (Lévi-Strauss, 1973, p. 73) and not simply in isolation. They are structures of relation as part of a system of relations. This functional interrelation between both spaces as system conditions allows for malleability and movement between these contrasting spaces, where increase in one can bring decrease in the other.

Relative Differences between Diametric and Concentric Spatial Systems: Mirror Image Symmetry, Closure/Openness and Assumed Separation/Connection

Lévi-Strauss observed two key contrasts between concentric and diametric structured systems. Diametric space offers (i) a feature of mirror image symmetry (Lévi-Strauss, 1973). A mirror image is not an identical one but a left-right inversion of polar opposites, for example, hierarchies of good/bad, success/failure, powerful/powerless (Downes, 2013). Diametric spaces are (ii) relatively more closed and boundaried than the more interactive with background and open concentric spatial systems. For concentric systems 'its frame of reference is always the environment ... In a diametric system ... virgin land constitutes an irrelevant element; the moieties are defined by their opposition to each other, and the apparent symmetry of their closed structure creates the illusion of a closed system' (Lévi-Strauss, 1963, p. 152).

In geographical thought on space, Massey (2005, p. 189) seeks a 'spatio-temporality which is open, through an open-ended temporality ... a spatiality that is both multiple and not closed ... always in the process of construction'. Concentric and diametric space is not a claim for an untenable absolute space openness, as a kind of blank page of empty possibility, that Massey could be interpreted as seeking here. However, Massey (2005, p. 165) seeks a more nuanced approach to space than one of simple flat openness versus closure: 'the issue is not bounded or unbounded in itself; not a simple opposition between spatial openness and spatial closure'. Massey (2005, p. 95) seeks an understanding that goes beyond simple binary oppositions between openness and closure, 'neither hermetic closure nor a world composed only of flow'. The interplay between concentric and diametric spatial systems offers a relative openness and closure, while also retaining a conception of openness that includes boundaries in its concentric expansive mode of assumed connection with background.

Characterising such concentric spatial systems as relatively more fluid ones (Downes, 2012), a further contrast has been identified (iii): a concentric spatial relation between poles is one of assumed connection, of mutual overlap around a common centre, a co-centre; in contrast, any interaction between diametrically oppositional poles is one of assumed separation and splitting (Downes, 2009, 2013). Though Lévi-Strauss did not explicitly highlight this difference, it is evident that the inner and outer poles of concentric structures are more fundamentally attached to each other than diametric structures. Both concentric poles coexist in the same space so that the outer circle overlaps the space of the inner one. The outer circle surrounds and contains the inner circle. In contrast, diametric oppositional realms are both basically detached and can be further smoothly detached from the other. A concentric relation assumes connection between its parts and any separation is on the basis of assumed connection, whereas diametric opposition assumes separation and any connection between the parts is on the basis of this assumed separation (Downes, 2009, 2013).

Reconstructing Diametric Spatial Mirror Image Symmetries in a Shift towards Concentric Spaces of Inclusion: Beyond Good/Bad Blame and Above/Below Hierarchy and Splitting Cultures in Education

Nurture rooms, as a key feature of Cooper's work (e.g. Cefai & Cooper, 2011; Cooper et al., 2001), offer spaces that are the epitome of concentric spatial systems of assumed connection, offering a trust, safety and emotional nurturance in school settings. A concentric spatial relation is a structure of inclusion compared to a diametric spatial structure of exclusion. In Bachelard's (1964, p. 212) words, pertinent to diametric space, 'simple geometrical opposition becomes tinged with aggressivity'. Nurture rooms take away an atmosphere of distrust and fractured relations, in other words, a diametric splitting of space into an oppositional atmosphere or climate of relations. In the words of the European Education and Training Expert Panel (2019, p. 71), 'creating concentric spaces, which will bring people together, can create feelings of social and emotional belonging'. This is a key concern of Cooper's (2008a) with regard to fostering student 'attachment' to school.

Such attachment can be construed here as developing concentric relational spaces of belonging, where students feel connected with school through supportive peer and teaching relationships. Attachment as a specifically spatial concept encompasses its loss as detachment in diametric spatial assumed separation and splitting, as well as ambivalence combining both love and hate, tender passivity and active hostility (Freud, 1926), as part of a mirror image inversion as a diametric structure (Downes, 2003, 2012). Space can amplify Cooper's concerns with attachment to school, involving concentric relational spaces and its loss as diametric spatial relations, of detachment, splitting and ambivalence leading to students' experiences of being an outsider in school. Concentric polarities in space offer a different, more connective model of inside-outside relation than one framed as diametric spatial conditions of rigid juxtaposition.

Cooper's work offers uncompromising accounts of the need to challenge old style communicative practices still adopted by some teachers, based on diametric oppositional spaces of fear and public embarrassment of students, what Cooper (2008a, p. 6) describes as 'problematic relationships with teachers'. Cooper (2008a, p. 6) recognises this as both a macrosystem societal flaw and microsystem school *lacuna* in communication, treating this wider 'concern with the failure of adult society, particularly as reflected in schools, to recognise and meet the emotional needs of young people'.

Cefai and Cooper's (2010, pp. 116–118) review of a number of small scale, Maltese studies with secondary students identified authoritarian teaching as a central issue, emerging from students' voices: 'One of the most common and frequently mentioned grievances by the students across the eight [Maltese] studies was the perceived lack of understanding and support by the classroom teachers. The students felt humiliated and inadequate when teachers shouted at them in front of their peers, ignored them or refused to listen to their views' In a forthright manner, Cefai and Cooper (2010, p. 188) highlight a pervasive theme of 'he autocratic and rigid behaviour management approach adopted by many teachers in their response to misbehaviour. Their blaming and punitive approach was seen in many cases as leading to an exacerbation of the problem ... It looks ... that perceived victimisation by teachers was more prevalent and had more impact than victimisation and bullying by peers'. These accounts criticising a diametric spatially imbued blame culture of good/bad students presaged the subsequent concerns with students' wellbeing raised in the WHO (2012) international survey of students' experiences in school, where the WHO explicitly raised concerns with teachers' public humiliation of pupils who perform poorly.

The European Education and Training Expert Panel (2019) recommends:

> The need to improve the relational and physical spaces in schools. This focuses on reconfiguring spaces in and around schools to provide safe spaces and relational spaces of belonging as a whole school approach ... Diametric oppositional spatial systems divide into us versus them, "good" students versus "bad" students, rigid "above/below" hierarchies. Such diametric splits in communication can lead to student fear of asking teachers questions. A contrasting concentric space is one in which both concentric poles are in assumed connection with each other around a common centre, offering a web of connectivity for inclusion. (p. 64)

Cefai and Cooper's (2010) emphasis on students' voices is tantamount to a dismantling of a diametric structured spatial hierarchy of above/below, where teachers are placed above and students below. This is not to instantiate a reverse diametric spatial hierarchy, where teachers are simply subservient to students. A different relational space is needed.

Concentric relational space manifests such a reconfiguration of relational spatial conditions. Concentric space offers a relation that allows for distinction between an inner and outer pole, while retaining an underlying connection; in other words, distinctions between teachers and students can be retained in concentric spatial relation (Downes, 2013), while doing so on the basis of an assumed connection of mutual trust and respect. As Cefai et al. (2021, p. 55) highlight, 'Diametric, oppositional spaces hinder trust and a sense of belonging, requiring a transition towards the concentric systems of relational space required to underpin whole-school assessment of SEE'. A reform agenda advocating students' voices, building on the UN Convention on the Rights of the Child, requires such voices to be given a concentric spatial-relational background of assumed connection (Downes, 2013) to ensure that they can be listened to and expressed in a climate of trust.

Spatial Concerns with Diametric Top-Down Hierarchy and Blank Space Monistic Reduction in Curricular Reform

Cooper (2008a) raises concerns with teachers' agency regarding the English National Curriculum's standards agenda. He highlights:

> The chief problem with these so-called reforms is that they have come to be experienced as a straitjacket that has reduced the role of the teacher from that of an innovator and interpreter of curricula to that of an implementer of a prescribed curriculum. (p. 16)

A Spatial Turn towards Concentric Systems of Inclusion   75

Cooper here offers an implicitly spatial hermeneutic role for the teacher to challenge their displacement into the passive pole of a diametric mirror image spatial opposition of active/passive, above/below.

A straitjacket is a constriction of space. Likewise authoritarian fear-based teaching congeals relational space into a closure of fear and division. Both express diametric spatial systems of relation. Cooper (2008a, p. 17) addresses not only students' fears but also those of teachers, referring to 'a climate of fear and aversion to risk' in teaching in England. He raises concerns with a policy and cultural climate where, 'Schools and teachers fear being publicly "named and shamed" if they step outside the limits of government guidelines – even when they believe the guidelines to be flawed'. Cooper challenges a top-down hierarchical movement that rests on a diametric spatial assumption to flatten education into a monistic reduction of schools and teachers to passive implementers, as technocrats who are mere instruments.

Diametric Space as a Precondition for Reification in Systems: Concerns for Commodification of Social and Emotional Education

In addition to concern with reification of teachers as mere instruments for curricular implementation (Cooper, 2008a), Cooper (2007, p. 21) describes 'the progressive commodification of UK higher education', while recognising that 'the current drift towards commodification is not confined to the domain of higher education. Similar developments are apparent across a range of hitherto public services', where he foregrounds the example of the UK National Health Service. Cooper invokes a concept of commodification processes in higher education as a relational system, though not specifically one in spatial terms:

> The unique extent to which commodified processes of education comprise an iterative and highly mutually interdependent relationship between students as buyers and

universities as sellers, in which both buyers and sellers must be very active participants to achieve a successful outcome, has been noted. (Cooper, 2007, p. 27)

Cooper's commodification concerns here are targeted at higher education, though they may also invite further questioning for early years, primary and postprimary education systems.

Two commingled aspects to commodification must be distinguished, at least to some degree. One identifies the commercial aspect of private interests seeking to engage in education for profit. A background aspect here is that commodification also involves a reification of education into packaged products, a dehumanising process of rendering education an object, an alienating process of loss of subjectivity in a process of objectification. It is this second background aspect to commodification that will be focused on here as spatial system conditions.

Diametric spatial relation is a standing opposite; the diametric poles are opposite each other. An object is in German, a *Gegenstand*, a standing against, which gives expression to objectification as a diametric oppositional relation, a distanciation between subject and object in Ricoeur's (1981) words. Fromm (1962, p. 149) develops this point, 'I – the observer – stand against my "ob-ject" … in German, Gegenstand = "counterstand"'. Diametric poles exemplify such ob-jectification and reification as they counterstand, juxtaposed against each other in opposition; a spatial precondition for objectification is diametric space. Massey's (2005, p. 52) phrase is apt here, 'to differentiate them counterpositionally one against the other' in the construction of the other. It is movement between contrasting spaces of diametric 'side-by-side' and concentric 'alongside' structures of relation that offers a perspective on change to reified systems. The rigid boundaries from background express the closed system of diametric space. They are prior spatial preconditions framing relations.

A spatial turn raises concerns with commodification of SEE in various guises of diametric space. It serves as a cautionary note towards summative assessment of SEE, where a diametric spatial winner/loser performativity might occur in SEE, an issue raised also in Cefai et al. (2021). Likewise, a concern with SEE as taking place as a diametric closed spatial system of rigidly prescribed outcomes that do not start from where the individual student is at, including a closure of prepackaged programmes in the SEE domain that do not adapt to individual differences and contexts, is part of a spatial questioning here. This is allied with critique of commercialisation of prepackaged SEE programmes.

Rigid SEE curricula that excise students' voices and specific life experiences operate within the diametric space of mirror image hierarchy between those with and without power in education. Top-down imposition of outcomes and prescribed skills risk not only a splitting from students' voices as part of a diametric spatial process and agenda to render the student passive, they also risk entering the terrain of SEE as social control, as mere cultural conditioning to create students as a 'cultural dope' (Garfinkel, 1967). The cross-culturally observed concentric spaces offer an antidote to such diametric spatial flattening of SEE into students as dehumanised automatons, what Fromm (1957) describes as merely prescribed 'personality packages'.

This spatial interrogation with diametric space as a process of reification in education recognises the potential for all areas, including SEE, to become alienated through this process. In doing so, this is not to accept the inevitability of SEE as an instrument of social control and conformity, as Ecclestone and Hayes (2009) tend to do. This critical spatial inquiry offers a path to scrutinise malleability of reified systems, as a corollary of commodification through diametric spatial features, including closure and a split non-interaction with background as an 'iron cage' (Weber, 1930, p. 181) around experience.

Diametric and Concentric Spaces of Experience as System Interactions; Key Spatial Conditions for Agency in a Biopsychosocial Framework for Psychological Development

Cooper's (2008b, p. 461) emphasis on a biopsychosocial framework of understanding recognises the need to reconceptualise beyond simple oppositional poles, while criticising 'the unhelpful polarity that is sometimes stated in terms of biological versus social explanations for learning and behavioural problems'. Challenge to simple polarity is again fertile ground for a further spatial interrogation as a shift from diametric spaces of opposition.

Experience has lain somewhat dormant as an active limb mediating between genetic and environmental factors influencing child development. There is increasing recognition of the need to avoid simplistic models of genetic determinism that overlook key enabling or hindering conditions from the environment (Gottlieb, 2002; Greene, 2014). Yet even those that invoke terminology of experience for development as part of an interactive understanding between genes and environment (Gottlieb & Halpern, 2002) still remain within highly limited conceptions of experience as agency.

Cooper (2008a, p. 462) expands on his position to highlight 'erroneous assumptions', such as 'that we have to choose between biomedical and environmental explanations for learning difficulties because they are incompatible'. Without entering the terrain of this debate on the overdiagnosis of ADHD, Cooper's wider point on the importance of embracing a biopsychosocial framework of understanding can be amplified also in spatial terms of concentric and diametric spatial systems. Recognising a broader view of causality as bidirectional coaction, in challenging reduction of psychological explanation to one level of explanation such as the genetic (resonant with Cooper's 2008b position), Gottlieb and Halpern (2002, p. 428) emphasise interactional dimensions for psychological phenomena: 'It is the particular combinations of environmental and genetic factors, and probably the timing of their coaction, that promote specific pathological outcomes'. This systemic recognition challenges a blank space role for genes. However, this does not add a conception of experience or experiential agency of the individual as a mediating factor, despite appeal to conceptions of experience.

Experience is envisaged in four different roles – anatomical, physiological, psychological and behavioural development – and as 'a relational term' (Gottlieb & Halpern, 2002, p. 423). That the very same term is employed for rats and humans – experience – attests to the poverty of this concept of experience. Experience is typically meant to mean events, such as '"postnatal handling" of rat pups (brief separation from their mother in the preweaning period)' (p. 428) rather than as an actively shaping experiential agency. In discussing early stressors in sensitising physiological systems in humans, the experiential reaction to the stressor is treated as experience, where 'like the animal models [of physiological reaction to stress] ... experience (i.e. coaction) can result in pathological outcomes across levels of a developmental system' (Gottlieb & Halpern, 2002, p. 429). A focus on experience resonant with a resilience focus interrogates the potential active response of the individual to these external stressor events and beyond physiological responses, though experience does appear to be treated, if equivalent to coaction, as a process where 'coactional processes' can cross levels of the developmental system (Gottlieb & Halpern, 2002, p. 429). Interpreted thus, experience as a relational spatial system can be a lost limb of the coactional processes mediating levels, to build on Gottlieb and Halpern (2002), while recognising that this is a broadening of Gottlieb's (1976, 2002) deliberately narrowed conception of experience.

Space is an active system as a purveyor of emotions, whether oppositional hostility and detachment of distrust in diametric space, or assumed connection, care and compassion (Downes, 2022b) of concentric space. Space also overcomes Cartesian splits between reason and emotion, where key cognitive constructs such as good/bad, norm/other, above/below hierarchy, love/hate, ingroup/outgroup are diametrically structured in spatial terms (Downes, 2020a). This can support an argument not only for a wider holistic conception of experience, encompassing interwoven emotions and cognitions, but to do so in concrete spatial terms as spatial systems. Experience is directly adverted to by early Bronfenbrenner's (1979) inclusion of phenomenology as a concern within his concentric ecological systems model. However, Bronfenbrenner's experiential concerns with phenomenology require further extension, including regarding his later biopsychosocial ecological systems framework (Bronfenbrenner & Evans, 2000). This amplification is not only in the relation to the various system levels for individuals' agency but also to treat experience in spatial systemic terms as interacting with other system levels. Experience as a spatial system of relations offers a distinctive, though related, system level to the macro–exo–meso–micro–chronosystem levels identified by Bronfenbrenner (1979, 2000).

Gottlieb's (2002, p. 163) review of gene-environment interaction in animals offers key insights for understanding experience as (a) supporting conditions for genetic processes and (b) part of a system, where 'the concept used most frequently to designate coactions at the organismic level of functioning is experience: experience is thus a relational term'. On this view, experience is relational as part of a system of interactions that includes genes. It is treated as 'interactive activity' (Gottlieb, 2002, p. 163) both for intrinsic relations within the organism and extrinsic ones (organism to organism, or organism to environment). Drawing on a wealth of research examples on experiential conditions as responding to the environment, such as warm temperatures to shock fruit fly larvae; developing rodent and chick brains in response to environmental input of nutrition and sensorimotor experience, including social isolation and environmental enrichment; mallard duck embryos hearing their own vocalisations; and chicks' sight of their own toes in the first days after hatching, Gottlieb's (2002) review develops an argument for experience as part of a wider interactional system. However, it does not treat such experience in spatial systemic terms.

The movement of interplay between concentric and diametric spaces as malleable contingent conditions of experience offers a domain of relevance, as a hypothesis to explain how experience can be potentially active supporting conditions to change the interactive dynamic of environmental-genetic determinism (Downes, 2020a). Though Lévi-Strauss did not bridge these structures to individual phenomenology, concentric and diametric spaces can apply to experiential domains, including personal identity, resilience, projections, obsessional neurosis, attachment and psychosis (Downes, 2012, 2020a). As spatial features of experience as preconditions supporting causal trajectories arising from environmental-genetic developmental chain reactions, this domain of concentric and diametric spaces structuring individual phenomenology offers a mediating discourse between phenomenology and causal explanations in developmental and educational psychology; it renders both experiential and causal levels more commensurable.

Conclusion

This chapter has argued that a critical spatial systems framework focusing on concentric and diametric spaces offers a cross culturally relevant lens for synthesising and expanding diverse strands of Cooper's interdisciplinary work, with regard to themes of social and emotional education, nurture rooms, overcoming fear and promoting agency, challenging commodification of education and the need for a biopsychosocial framework. Agency is understood as active experiential movements between malleable diametric and concentric spatial conditions in a system, as part of gene-experience-environment interactions for a broadened critical spatial biopsychosocial model. Agency is embedded in movement between concentric and diametric systems, to promote inclusion and challenge hierarchy, othering, discrimination and exclusions (Downes, 2020a). This treats these spaces not only as structures but as directional processes in mutual interactive tension. This active role for systems as spatial movements, including as a system of experience, challenges traditional Western Cartesian conceptions of space as empty, echoed also in Locke's *tabula rasa*.

A critical spatial lens is being proposed in order to interrogate power and reification, thematic aspects underplayed by Bronfenbrenner's ecological systems theory, though of direct concern for Cooper. As part of a concentric spatial turn building on Cooper's work, future questions of concern include reification processes for SEE examined as diametric spatial systems and system blockages in education, as well as the need for fresh concentric spaces for connection such as school gardens for SEE, as well as outdoor education spaces for social and emotional development. This spatial reading offers concretisation of system critiques in terms of diametric spaces and opportunities to shift from these towards specific concentric relational spatial systems as directions of relative connection and openness.

References

Bachelard, G. (1964/1994). *The poetics of space*. Beacon Press.
Bronfenbrenner, U. (1979). *The ecology of human development*. Harvard University Press.
Bronfenbrenner, U., & Evans, G. W. (2000). Developmental science in the 21st century: Emerging questions, theoretical models, research designs and empirical findings. *Social Development, 9*(1), 115–125.
Cefai, C., & Cooper, P. (2010). Students without voices: The unheard accounts of secondary school students with social, emotional and behaviour difficulties. *European Journal of Special Needs Education, 25*(2), 183–198.
Cefai, C., & Cooper, P. (2011). The introduction of nurture groups in Maltese schools: A method of promoting inclusive education. *British Journal of Special Education, 38*, 65–72.
Cefai, C., Downes, P., & Cavioni, V. (2021). *A formative, inclusive, whole-school approach to the assessment of social and emotional education in the EU*. Publications Office of the European Union/EU Bookshop.
Cooper, P. (2007). Knowing your 'Lemons': Quality uncertainty in UK higher education. *Quality in Higher Education, 13*(1), 19–29.
Cooper, P. (2008a). Nurturing attachment to school: Contemporary perspectives on social, emotional, and behavioural difficulties. *Pastoral Care in Education, 26*(1), 13–22.
Cooper, P. (2008b). Like alligators bobbing for poodles? A critical discussion of education, ADHD and the biopsychosocial perspective. *Journal of Philosophy of Education, 42*(3–4), 457–474.
Cooper, P., Arnold, R., & Boyd, E. (2001). The effectiveness of Nurture Groups: Preliminary research findings. *British Journal of Special Education, 28*(4), 160–166.
Descartes, R. (1954). *Descartes: Philosophical writings* (Trans. E. Anscombe & P. T. Geach). Nelson.
Downes, P. (2003). Cross-cultural structures of concentric and diametric dualism in Lévi-Strauss' structural anthropology: Structures of relation underlying the self and ego relation. *Journal of Analytical Psychology, 48*(1), 47–81.
Downes, P. (2009). Prevention of bullying at a systemic level in schools: Movement from cognitive and spatial narratives of diametric opposition to concentric relation. In S. R. Jimerson, S. M. Swearer, & D. L. Espelage (Eds), *Handbook of bullying in schools: An international perspective* (pp. 517–533). Routledge.

Downes, P. (2011). The neglected shadow: Some European perspectives on emotional supports for early school leaving prevention. *International Journal of Emotional Education, 3*(2), 3–39.
Downes, P. (2012). *The primordial dance: Diametric and concentric spaces in the unconscious world.* Peter Lang.
Downes, P. (2013). Developing a framework and agenda for students' voices in the school system across Europe: From diametric to concentric relational spaces for early school leaving prevention. *European Journal of Education, 48*(3), 346–362.
Downes, P. (2020a). *Reconstructing agency in developmental and educational psychology: Inclusive systems as concentric space.* Routledge.
Downes, P. (2020b). *Concentric space as a life principle beyond Schopenhauer, Nietzsche and Ricoeur: Inclusion of the other.* Routledge.
Ecclestone, K., & Hayes, D. (2009). *The dangerous rise of therapeutic education.* Routledge.
European Commission, European Education and Training Expert Panel. (2019). *Issue paper on inclusion and citizenship.* Education and Training ET 2020.
Ferrare, J. J., & Apple, M. W. (2010). Spatializing critical education: Progress and cautions. *Critical Studies in Education, 51,* 209–221.
Freud, S. (1926). Inhibitions, symptoms and anxiety. In J. Strachey & A. Freud (Eds), *The standard edition of the complete psychological works of Sigmund Freud* (pp. 77–175). Hogarth Press.
Fromm, E. (1957). *The art of loving.* Harper & Brothers.
Fromm, E. (1962/1990). *Beyond the chains of illusion: My encounter with Marx and Freud.* Continuum.
Garfinkel, H. (1967). *Studies in ethnomethodology.* Prentice Hall.
Gottlieb, G. (1976). The roles of experience in the development of behavior and the nervous system. *Studies on the Development of Behavior and the Nervous System, 3,* 25–54.
Gottlieb, G. (2002). *Individual development and evolution: The genesis of novel behaviour.* Psychology Press.
Gottlieb, G., & Halpern, C. T. (2002). A relational view of causality in normal and abnormal development. *Development and Psychopathology, 14,* 421–435.
Greene, S. (2014). *The psychological development of girls and women: Rethinking change in time* (2nd rev. edn). Routledge.
Jung, C. G. (1936/1985). Individual dream symbolism in relation to alchemy. In C. G. Jung (Ed.), *Dreams.* Ark.
Leach, E. (1965/2000). Claude Lévi-Strauss: Anthropologist and philosopher. In S. Hugh-Jones & J. Laidlaw (Eds), *The essential Edmund Leach* (Vol. I, Anthropology and society). Yale University Press.
Lévi-Strauss, C. (1962/1966). *The savage mind* (Trans. G. Weidenfeld). Nicolson Ltd.

Lévi-Strauss, C. (1963). *Structural anthropology*: *Vol. 1* (Trans. C. Jacobsen & B. Grundfest Schoepf). Allen Lane: Penguin Books. Lévi-Strauss, C. (1973/1977). *Structural anthropology: Vol. 2* (Trans. M. Layton). Penguin Books.

Mannion, G. (2007). Going spatial, going relational: Why 'listening to children' and children's participation needs reframing. *Discourse: Studies in the Cultural Politics of Education*, *28*, 405–420.

Massey, D. (2005*). For space.* Sage Publications.

Ricoeur, P. (1981). *Hermeneutics and the human sciences* (Trans. J. B. Thompson). Cambridge University Press.

Weber, M. (1930). *The protestant ethic and the spirit of capitalism*. Allen & Unwin.

World Health Organisation (WHO). (2012). Social determinants of health and wellbeing among young people. *Health Behaviour in School-Aged Children (HBSC) Study: International report from the 2009/2010 survey*. WHO.

VALERIA CAVIONI AND GIUSI ANTONIA TOTO

6 Exploring Pre-service Special Education Teachers' Self-Perceptions in Addressing Students' Academic, Social, and Emotional Needs

Introduction

This chapter explores the perceptions of pre-service teachers in special education and their essential contribution to shaping the trajectory of inclusive education in the years to come. With a profound connection to the work of Paul Cooper, a luminary in the field of student engagement and inclusion, our study investigates the essence of what it means to prepare the educators of tomorrow for students with special educational needs. Paul Cooper's extensive body of work, grounded over decades of research, has been focused on the multifaceted needs of students with diverse educational needs. In this chapter, we connected the research and experiences offered by Professor Cooper's work with the knowledge and practical implications of teacher pre-service education raised by our findings, fostering a holistic understanding of the intricate interplay that unites teachers' identity, inclusion, and student support.

Background

In contemporary education, the role of teachers has been extended far beyond the conventional boundaries of disseminating academic knowledge; indeed, teaching involves fostering the comprehensive and healthy development of students (Cavioni & Grazzani, 2023; Cefai & Cavioni,

2014; Conte et al., 2023). With an increased emphasis on addressing the multifaceted psychological needs of students at school, educators are now asked to tailor their practice to provide academic, social, and emotional support, thereby fostering inclusive school environments for all learners (Aldridge & McChesney, 2018; Cefai & Cooper, 2009; Toto, 2021). The paradigm of inclusive education has garnered increasing attention for its emphasis on ensuring equitable opportunities for all students, particularly those with special educational needs (Cefai & Cooper, 2009; Cooper, 2011).

In this context, several studies underlined the key role of the teacher-student relationship which constitutes a cornerstone of education, wielding a profound influence on students' mental health and academic achievements (Cavioni et al., 2017, 2021; Cefai et al., 2013; O'Connor et al., 2011). Establishing positive teacher-student relationships empowers educators to enhance students' sense of belonging and emotional security within the school environment. A trusting teacher-student relationship provides a secure base from which students can explore and manage their own emotions and develop social relationships with peers and adults that are crucial for both school and life success (Jennings & Greenberg, 2009; Limone & Toto, 2022; Mahoney et al., 2021).

The role of special education teachers is particularly linked with the quality of the relationships they establish with their students, especially for those who require additional support (Cooper & McIntyre, 1996; Murray & Pianta, 2007). Central to this endeavour is the essential education and consequent contribution of pre-service teachers, individuals poised on the threshold of embarking on their professional journeys (Ahsan et al., 2013; Nalipay et al., 2021). In this scenario, special education teachers emerge as potent change agents, wielding the capacity to model the forthcoming school settings with their distinct viewpoints, approaches, and innovative strategies. Their presence not only holds the promise of enriching inclusive educational environments but also has the potential to deeply impact on the academic and psychological well-being of their students with special educational needs (Dickenson et al., 2016; Toto, 2021).

The perceptions of teachers of special education about themselves as professionals play a significant role in their teaching practices and effectiveness in the classroom (EADSNE, 2012; Saloviita, 2020). Attitudes and self-perceptions developed during teacher education programs tend to be resistant to alteration if not entirely immutable (Ahsan et al., 2013; Dunne, 2019; Kane et al., 2002; Richardson, 1996). Consequently, more research is needed to ensure that upon completing teachers' education programs, pre-service teachers possess the adequate disposition to engage in inclusive practices as prospective teachers in the classroom (Aiello et al., 2018). The present study sought to investigate the self-perception of pre-service teachers in special education on their future profession and to identify their positive and negative capacities and attitudes in addressing the academic, social, and emotional needs of students with special educational needs.

Method

Participants

The participants in this study were 134 special pre-service teachers (103 female; mean age = 38,18, sd = 8,25; min age = 22; max age = 59) enrolled in a professional course for high school special education teachers at the University of Foggia, in Italy. Participants were informed about the purpose of the study and the voluntary nature of their participation. Informed consent was obtained before their participation.

A significant number of the participants (n = 96) held a master's degree; sixteen possessed a high school diploma, fifteen a post-lauream degree or PhD and a few participants (n = 6) obtained the bachelor's degree as their highest completed level of education. The participants came from different academic backgrounds mainly related to education, psychology, and humanities fields. Most participants (n = 115) had very little experience (zero up to three years) in formal teaching roles prior to their enrolment in this teacher education program. The remaining had a longer teaching experience ranging from four to thirteen years. Most participants predominantly originated from southern Italian regions, with a notable concentration from the Puglia region, where the University of Foggia is located.

Procedure

The study employed a qualitative research design to explore the pre-service teachers' self-perception as future educators in the context of inclusive education. The data collection was structured into four distinct phases. In the initial phase, the participants were engaged in a self-portrait activity designed to elicit their self-concept and capacity as future teachers to address the complex needs of students with special educational needs. Participants were provided with art supplies, including paper, coloured pencils, markers, and other artistic materials. They were encouraged to consider various aspects of their professional identity, including their roles, emotions, attitudes, and expectations they believed were essential in supporting students with diverse educational needs. This individual self-portrait activity allowed participants to express their internal concepts and aspirations in a non-verbal, visual format.

In the second phase of the study, participants were directed to individually add a list of adjectives to their self-portraits. This was aimed to provide linguistic descriptors that aligned with the visual representations in their self-portraits, offering a deeper layer of insight into their self-concepts and serving to encapsulate the qualities and attributes they believed were integral to their perceived roles as future special educators. Importantly, these adjectives encompassed a spectrum of representations and emotions including both positive and negative connotations that reflected participants' feelings, self-representations, and even underlying concerns and fears. The collection of these adjectives, whether positive or negative, not only enriched the participants' self-portraits but also contributed to a more holistic exploration of their self-perceptions.

In the subsequent phase, participants were divided into small discussion groups, each consisting of ten to twelve individuals. Within these groups, they engaged in collaborative discussions to explore the qualitative insights derived from their self-portraits and the accompanying adjectives.

The small group format allowed for in-depth conversations, enabling participants to share their perspectives, interpretations, and reflections on their own self-concepts emerging from the self-portrait and individual adjectives activities.

Following the small group discussions, the study transitioned into a larger forum. Participants reconvened as a whole group, where they collectively shared their reflections from the small group interactions. In this open setting, they had the opportunity to offer insights, engage in cross-group comparisons, and share overarching themes that emerged from the discussions. This phase facilitated a comprehensive exploration of the diverse viewpoints and commonalities present within the sample.

Data Collection and Data Analysis Strategy

The researchers collected qualitative data from each phase, including individual self-portraits, individual lists of adjectives, small-group discussions, and collective reflections from the entire group discussion. These multiple data sources enriched the analysis by providing a multifaceted perspective on participants' self-perceptions. To ensure the authenticity and confidentiality of the data collected, participants were assured that their self-portraits and lists of adjectives would remain anonymous and used solely for research purposes.

The data collected from the various phases of data collection underwent a rigorous process of thematic analysis (Braun & Clarke, 2006). This type of analysis facilitated a comprehensive exploration of the data collected from the various phases of the study acknowledging the complexity of participants' self-perceptions and the dynamic interplay between their self-representations and emotional experiences, since the participants were also encouraged to select adjectives that resonated with their self-concept, and emotional responses to their envisioned roles.

Data analysis involved two experienced researchers to enhance the inter-rater reliability and to minimise the risk of personal biases affecting the interpretation of themes, a crucial aspect of ensuring consistency and accuracy in the analysis contributing to the validity of the findings. The involvement of two researchers enabled consensus building during the process of themes' identification and labelling. Through negotiation and discussions, a higher level of agreement was reached on the interpretation and categorisation of themes.

The process of thematic analysis involved different phases. The initial step involved immersing the researchers in the data collected from each phase. This process allowed the researchers to gain a comprehensive understanding of participants' self-portraits, adjectives, and the discussions that unfolded during the small-group and whole-group interactions. Transcriptions of group discussions and written reflections were reviewed to establish familiarity with the contents. The data were then systematically coded to identify recurring words, phrases, and patterns across the phases. For the self-portraits and adjectives, individual elements were coded to capture the qualities, emotions, and attributes participants described. Themes began to emerge as codes were grouped based on shared meanings. The small group discussions and whole group reflections were similarly coded to capture common ideas and insights. Themes were refined through a process of comparison and grouping. Codes were organised into potential themes that captured the essence of participants' self-perceptions, aspirations, and concerns. Finally, themes were named to encapsulate the essence of the data they represented. The connections between different phases of data collection were considered to understand how themes evolved and resonated across the diverse dataset. The researchers engaged in an interpretive process to derive meaningful insights from the identified themes. The interpretation was cross-referenced with the original data to ensure accuracy and alignment with participants' expressions.

Results

The inclusion of both positive and negative adjectives allowed participants to authentically convey the multifaceted nature of their self-identified qualities as well as their apprehensions as prospective teachers in special education. In particular, the utilization of adjectives with varying emotional tones provided a deeper layer of insight into their self-conceptualisation. It illuminated the dichotomy between their aspirations and potential anxieties, fostering a more nuanced understanding of their readiness and emotional preparedness to address the academic, social, and emotional needs of students with special educational needs.

Overall, the resulting themes evoked feelings of care, protection and enthusiasm which were represented through positive adjectives. Indeed, many teachers depicted themselves as compassionate and dedicated educators committed to ensuring the success of their students. Others emphasised the desire to be a guide while fostering supportive and inclusive learning environments. Conversely, some teachers expressed concerns about potential challenges they might encounter, such as not being adequately trained in managing challenging behaviours or meeting individualised educational needs.

Through a comprehensive analysis of their self-portraits, accompanied by thoughtful adjectives, six distinct themes emerged, each offering a unique lens into the values, aspirations, qualities, and challenges that these aspiring educators envisioned.

Theme 1: Nurturing Presence

This category encompassed a wide spectrum of adjectives that collectively characterise teachers' perceived roles as caring educators. Participants expressed their intent to embody qualities that make their classrooms welcoming, loving, and friendly. They aspire to be reliable and available figures for their students, instilling a sense of trust and dependability. Participants envision themselves as passionate, charismatic, and understanding educators – qualities that are vital in creating an environment where students feel safe to express themselves and seek guidance. The frequently reported adjectives 'motivating', 'encouraging', 'caring' and 'reassuring' emphasise their commitment to inspire their students to pursue educational engagement and success. Furthermore, qualities such as being sensitive, empathic, and reassuring highlighted the teachers' dedication to addressing the social and emotional needs of their students. Figure

6.1 provides an example of the visual representation of one of the self-portraits drawn by a participant illustrating openness, genuineness, and care for the needs of the students. In this drawing, the teacher is depicted with an open and visible heart which serves as a powerful metaphor for the teacher's authenticity, caring, and empathy.

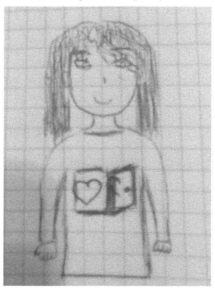

Figure 6.1. Self-portrait depicting a teacher's openness, caring and empathy

Another self-portrait (see Figure 6.2) offers a distinctive perspective on the role of a special educator as a careful, nurturing and attentive caretaker, akin to a gardener tending to the needs of a growing plant. In this artwork, the teacher is depicted beside a flourishing plant, mirroring the nurturing relationship between educator and students. This portrait captures a sense of patience, dedication, and responsibility as the teacher is shown tending to the plant's needs. The imagery speaks to the teachers' desire to foster an environment where each child's unique growth trajectory is cultivated with care, allowing students to flourish academically, socially, and emotionally.

This category summarises the educators' commitment to being attentive caregivers who provide essential nourishment for students' development as well as signal their intention to foster a caring foundation that

Pre-service Special Education Teachers' Self-Perceptions

enables students to flourish in an environment filled with attention and opportunities for growth.

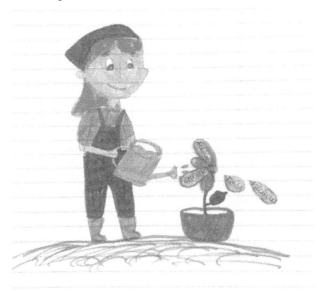

Figure 6.2. Self-portrait depicting the teacher as a gardener taking care of students' needs

Theme 2: Leaders Providing Guidance and Protection

This theme includes the qualities and attributes that teachers associate with their roles as educational leaders who serve as guides and sources of protection. The adjectives within this theme emphasise the teachers' dedication to assume the role of leader in both instructional and nurturing capacities. More specifically, the adjectives reflect participants' aspirations to be not only educators but also trusted guides, supervisors, and protectors of their students. This underscores the teachers' intent to take on the role of a landmark – a dependable reference point – within their students' educational journeys. Indeed, examples of types of adjectives provided by the teachers included terms such as 'landmark', 'guide', 'leader', and 'supervisor'. Figure 6.3 represents a self-portrait depicting the teacher as a lighthouse radiating light onto the life and development of students, with a student depicted at three different stages of her school life. This artwork captures the essence of the teacher's aspiration to be a guiding beacon, illuminating the path of learning and personal development for their students, as they progress through the various stages of their educational journey.

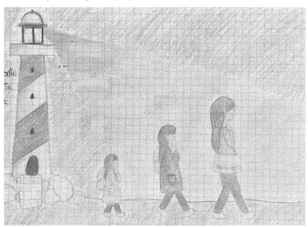

Figure 6.3. Self-portrait depicting the teacher as a lighthouse to supervise and guide the students across age stages in their education

The teacher's aspiration to be a reliable source of guidance, steering their students toward educational and personal success across the years has been also frequently represented by the metaphor of a compass (e.g. Figure 6.4). Indeed, the compass' representation of cardinal directions, namely North, East, South, and West, translates metaphorically into the teacher's commitment to provide comprehensive and extended guidance. Just as the compass ensures travellers remain on the right path, teachers aspire to safeguard that their students safely navigate the complexities of learning with clear purposes. Furthermore, such self-portraits of teachers as compasses evoke the idea of consistency and reliability as they aim to be a constant and dependable presence in their students' educational journeys.

Pre-service Special Education Teachers' Self-Perceptions 95

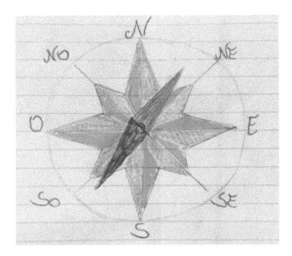

Figure 6.4. Self-portrait depicting the teacher as a compass providing directions to students

Theme 3: Joyful Engagement and Playful Interaction

This theme condenses the qualities and attributes that teachers associate with their roles as educators who infuse imagination, fun, and humour into the learning experiences. The adjectives in this category highlight the teachers' commitment to fostering a lively, enjoyable, joyful, and creatively stimulating educational setting. Examples of adjectives by the teachers included being 'cheerful', 'self-deprecating', 'funny', and 'ironic'. This theme also emphasises the teachers' intent to incorporate creativity and imaginative exploration in their pedagogy to cultivate a school environment where students feel welcomed, valued, and eager to participate. Figure 6.5 depicts a teacher holding a magic wand. This artwork symbolises the teacher's aspiration to be a 'magician' of learning, infusing the educational experience with elements of wonder and imagination. The magic wand embodies the teacher's intention to create enchanting and captivating learning experiences, much like a magician conjuring moments of awe and delight. Just as a magician mesmerises an audience, these teachers aspire to captivate their students' attention, sparking curiosity and excitement in the process.

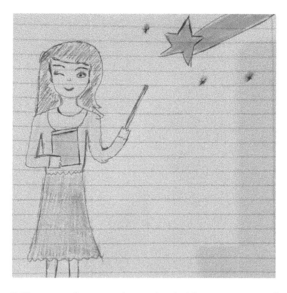

Figure 6.5. Self-portrait depicting the teacher holding a magic wand to enhance imagination and spark students' interest and participation

Theme 4: Professional Integrity and Ethical Practice

This theme summarises the qualities and attributes that participants associate with their roles as educators committed to upholding democratic principles, fairness, and ethical conduct in their practice. The adjectives in this theme collectively emphasise the teachers' dedication to maintain a balanced, fair, and impartial educational environment. The adjectives emphasise the participants' commitment to create a serene and equitable learning atmosphere. This theme also reflects the participants' dedication to ensure that correct information is disseminated, equitable opportunities are provided, and diverse viewpoints are acknowledged. The adjectives highlight the teachers' commitment to cultivate an atmosphere free from bias. Examples of suggestions by teachers included being 'democratic', 'fair', 'balanced', and 'impartial'. The emphasis on qualities such as calmness, fairness, patience, and impartiality reflected the participants' intent to create a serene and inclusive space where all students, especially those with SENs, feel comfortable expressing their thoughts, engaging in thoughtful discussions, and learning without fear of judgement.

As an illustration of this theme, we have included a drawing of a teacher who depicted himself seated beside a river, exuding calmness, and surrounded by moving leaves (Figure 6.6). The teacher's calm presence amidst the movement of leaves represents his aspiration to maintain equanimity and his ability to remain fair even during challenges. Hence, the juxtaposition of the teacher's calmness against the moving leaves reflects the notion of being a stable landmark amid the fluctuations of classroom dynamics. Furthermore, the flowing river symbolises the continuous changes that are part of school life as well as the flow of knowledge, experiences, and diverse perspectives in the educational journey.

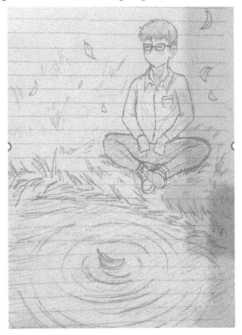

Figure 6.6. Self-portrait depicting the teacher's ability to build an atmosphere of serenity and equity

Theme 5: Supportive Catalysts for Thriving

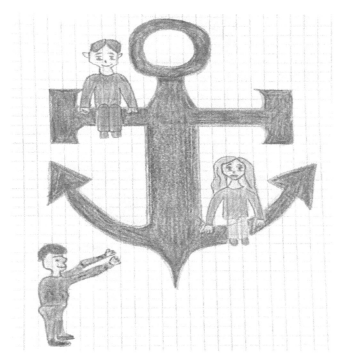

Figure 6.7. Self-portrait illustrating the teacher as an anchor providing stability and assistance to students

This theme refers to teachers' roles as facilitators of empowerment and overall well-being. The adjectives underline the teachers' commitment to being lifelines of assistance, anchors of stability, and tools for enabling their students to thrive and flourish despite their difficulties. 'Lifeline', 'support', and 'helper' were some of the adjectives used by the participants. These participants envision themselves as lifelines that offer essential support, anchors that provide stability, and tools that enable their students to thrive in all aspects of their lives. Some of the collected self-portraits referred to the image of an anchor. Accordingly, Figure 6.7 portrays a teacher as an anchor, with students with special needs finding support in the teacher as a landmark. The anchor embodies the teacher's intention to be a steadfast source of support, providing stability, empowerment, instructional and emotional support for students with SENs who may face unique challenges.

Theme 6: Self-Doubt and Emerging Growth

This theme refers to the qualities and attributes that teachers associate with their self-perceived areas of vulnerability, inexperience, and areas for potential growth. While it is evident that some adjectives provided by teachers, such as 'anxious', 'fragile', 'insecure', 'inexperienced', and 'fearful of making mistakes', point to an acknowledgement of vulnerabilities, this signifies a deeper awareness of the emotional complexities inherent in teaching, particularly in managing students' behavioural issues or in adapting the curriculum to the students' individual needs. Moreover, this openness to recognise personal challenges also reflects the participants' dedication to self-improvement and their understanding that these challenges can be catalysts for growth and professional development. By acknowledging their anxieties, insecurities, and fears of making mistakes, they reveal their intent to confront vulnerabilities, viewing them as stepping stones towards self-improvement as well as an aspiration to address these difficulties, fostering their professional growth. Figure 6.8 illustrates a teacher holding a road sign with two possible directions symbolising the difficult choices and decisions that teachers may encounter during their careers. This drawing suggests the participant's introspective exploration of their professional journey, acknowledging the presence of uncertainties and the ongoing process of self-discovery and growth.

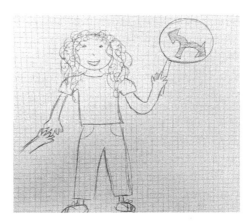

Figure 6.8. Self-portrait depicting the teacher holding a road sign with two possible directions

Discussion

In this study, we explored the self-perceptions of special education preservice teachers and the implications for their future roles as educators. By doing so, we hope to contribute to expanding the literature on teacher self-concept and its impact on future educational approaches in addressing students' needs, particularly those with special educational needs. Through a comprehensive thematic analysis, six compelling themes emerged, shedding light on the multifaceted dimensions of the participants' self-concepts and aspirations. The six themes – nurturing presence, leaders providing guidance and protection, joyful engagement and playful interaction, professional integrity and ethical practice, supportive catalysts for thriving, and self-doubt and emerging growth – offer deep insights into how these aspiring educators envision their roles.

To establish an understanding of the intricate ways in which these six themes intersect with the teachers' commitment to inclusive education, it is imperative to delve deeper into each theme's essence and how it aligns with the principles of fostering inclusive learning environments. We will now explore how these themes unfold within the context of educators' dedication to creating classrooms where all students, including those with SENs, are welcomed, valued, and empowered.

The theme named 'nurturing presence' resonates deeply with teachers' commitment to inclusive education. As educators envision themselves as sources of emotional guidance and safety, they inherently create an environment where all students, regardless of their backgrounds or abilities, feel valued, cared for, and included. This theme reflects the foundational role of teachers in fostering a sense of belonging, crucial for the success of inclusive classrooms (Cooper & Cefai, 2013). By being nurturing and supportive, these prospective teachers demonstrate a commitment to creating an inclusive atmosphere where every student's needs are met with care and understanding (Cooper & Tiknaz, 2007).

The theme 'Leaders providing guidance and protection' is also intricately connected with the participants' commitment to inclusive education. By viewing themselves as leaders who guide and protect their students' learning journeys, these educators embrace the responsibility of ensuring that each student has equitable access to education. Their leadership extends to advocating for inclusive practices, making adaptations, and promoting an environment where diversity is celebrated, and everyone's potential is realised. This theme underscores their dedication to advocating for the rights and needs of students with diverse abilities (Bradley-Levine, 2021).

The third theme 'Joyful engagement and playful interaction' highlights the participants' motivation to create inclusive classrooms that foster engagement and joy for all students. Educators who embody this theme recognise that joyful learning experiences transcend barriers and encourage active participation from every student (Fredrickson & Branigan, 2005). By infusing playfulness, imagination, and enthusiasm into their teaching, these educators promote a sense of inclusion where students with diverse abilities feel motivated to explore, learn, and collaborate. This theme reflects the participants' commitment to breaking down the traditional boundaries that might hinder the active participation of students with special needs, facilitating their engagement through a child-and special needs-friendly pedagogy.

The theme 'Professional integrity and ethical practice' underscores the participants' awareness of ethical attitudes and behaviours in inclusive education. By upholding professional integrity and ethical standards, educators ensure that all students are treated with respect and dignity. This theme reflects commitment to fairness, advocating for equitable opportunities, and challenging any discriminatory practices. The participants' commitment to ethical practices aligns with the principles of inclusive education, ensuring that the rights and well-being of all students, including those most vulnerable, are upheld (Athanases & de Oliveira, 2007).

The theme 'Supportive catalysts for thriving' embodies participants' commitment to foster an environment where every student can participate and thrive. As these seek to facilitate their students' growth, they are actively ensuring that all students, including those with special educational needs, have the necessary support and resources to succeed despite their challenges. Such a theme profoundly resonates with the concept of resilience – a quality that is paramount in nurturing students' ability to overcome challenges, adapt, and flourish in the face of adversity (Cavioni et al., 2018; Cefai et al., 2015; Höltge et al., 2021). This theme also emphasises the participant's commitment to provide personalised assistance, adapting instruction, and offering individualised pathways to success (Cooper, 2017). In doing so, they aim to create a learning environment where students are not only equipped with the necessary skills but are also fortified with the capacity to bounce back from setbacks and emerge stronger (Cefai et al., 2018; Grazzani et al., 2022; Martinsone et al., 2022).

The last theme, namely 'Self-doubt and emerging growth', reflects the prospective teachers' desire for continuous improvement. By acknowledging their own areas of uncertainty and vulnerability, they demonstrate willingness to learn from mistakes. Their commitment to self-improvement aligns with the evolving nature of inclusive education, where teachers must constantly adapt to meet the diverse needs of their students. This theme reflects their motivation to be responsive, reflective practitioners who continuously strive to enhance their abilities to create inclusive learning environments. It underlines the critical importance of fostering teacher preparedness for the challenges of the profession and the educators' own wellbeing (Lester et al., 2020; Toto & Limone, 2021). Thus, it is vital to acknowledge these capacities cannot develop and flourish without a foundation of personal well-being. Teachers who feel empowered and supported in their roles are more likely to be mentally healthy, and resilient, thus equipping them to effectively address the diverse students' needs, including those with special needs (Cavioni et al., 2023b). Recognising the challenges and complexities of teaching, these prospective teachers acknowledge the significance of their own mental health and wellbeing (Cavioni et al., 2020). This self-awareness can lead to the creation of a positive feedback loop where educators who prioritise their well-being are better equipped to provide the adequate support their students require (Cefai et al., 2022).

The exploration of special education pre-service teachers' self-perceptions and their alignment with the identified themes serves as evidence of the critical importance of preparing inclusive and caring educators. Teachers in special education need to be trained to foster a nurturing environment, provide leadership and guidance, engage students in enjoyable learning experiences, uphold ethical standards, support growth, and remain open to improvement. These qualities and capacities will ensure that teachers will play a pivotal role in ensuring that all students, regardless of their abilities or backgrounds, have access to quality education in inclusive settings.

Conclusion

This study contributed to the few previous existing literature on teachers' self-perception as special needs educators, an area that remains relatively underexplored despite its potential impact on teaching and learning (Aiello et al., 2018). Understanding how teacher self-perception may influence professional development can lead to the development of targeted interventions and support systems for teachers to enhance their effectiveness as educators. While this study provides valuable insights, it is not without limitations. The sample primarily represents a specific geographic region, potentially limiting the generalisability of findings to broader contexts. Additionally, the self-report nature of the data may introduce biases or social desirability effects. The thematic analysis, while robust, is subject to interpretation and subjectivity inherent to qualitative research. Building upon the foundation laid by this study, future researchers can explore how these self-perceptions may evolve as these pre-service teachers transition into their professional roles.

References

Ahsan, M. T., Deppeler, J. M., & Sharma, U. (2013). Predicting pre-service teachers' preparedness for inclusive education: Bangladeshi pre-service teachers' attitudes and perceived teaching-efficacy for inclusive education. *Cambridge Journal of Education*, *43*(4), 517–535.

Aiello, P., Pace, E. M., Dimitrov, D. M., & Sibilio, M. (2018). A study on the perceptions and efficacy towards inclusive practices of teacher trainees. *Italian Journal of Educational Research*, *19*, 13–28.

Aldridge, J. M., & McChesney, K. (2018). The relationships between school climate and adolescent mental health and wellbeing: A systematic literature review. *International Journal of Educational Research*, *1*(88), 121–145.

Athanases, S. Z., & de Oliveira, L. C. (2007). Conviction, confrontation, and risk in new teachers' advocating for equity. *Teaching Education*, *18*(2), 123–136.

Bradley-Levine, J. (2021). Examining teacher advocacy for full inclusion. *Journal of Catholic Education*, *24*(1), 62–82.

Braun, V., & Clarke, V. (2006). Using thematic analysis in psychology. *Qualitative Research in Psychology*, *3*(2), 77–101.

Cavioni, V., & Grazzani, I. (2023). *L'apprendimento sociale ed emotivo: Teorie e buone pratiche per promuovere la salute mentale a scuola*. Il Mulino.

Cavioni, V., Grazzani, I., & Ornaghi, V. (2017). Social and emotional learning for children with learning disability: Implications for inclusion. *International Journal of Emotional Education*, *9*(2), 100–109.

Cavioni, V., Grazzani, I., & Ornaghi, V. (2020). Mental health promotion in schools: A comprehensive theoretical framework. *International Journal of Emotional Education*, *12*(1), 65–82.

Cavioni, V., Grazzani, V., Ornaghi, V., Agliati, A., & Pepe, A. (2021). Adolescents' mental health at school: The mediating role of life satisfaction. *Frontiers in Psychology*, *12*, 720628. <https://doi.org/10.3389/fpsyg.2021.720628>.

Cavioni, V., Conte, E., Grazzani, I., Ornaghi, V., Cefai, C., Anthony, C., ... Pepe, A. (2023a). Validation of Italian students' self-ratings on the SSIS SEL brief scales. *Frontiers in Psychology, 14*, 1229653. <https://doi.org/10.3389/fpsyg.2023.1229653>.

Cavioni, V., Grazzani, V., Ornaghi, V., Agliati, A., Gandellini, S., Cefai, C., ... Conte, E. (2023b). A multi-component curriculum to promote teachers' mental health: Findings from the PROMEHS program. *International Journal of Emotional Education, 15*(1), 34–52.

Cavioni, V., Zanetti, M. A., Beddia, G., & Lupica Spagnolo, M. (2018). Promoting resilience: A European curriculum for students, teachers and families. In M. Wosnitza, F. Peixoto, S. Beltman, & C. Mansfield (Eds), *Resilience in education: Concepts, contexts and connections* (pp. 313–332). Springer International Publishing.

Cefai, C., Arlove, A., Duca, M., Galea, N., Muscat, M., & Cavioni, V. (2018). RESCUR surfing the waves: An evaluation of a resilience programme in the early years. *Pastoral Care in Education, 36*(3), 189–204.

Cefai, C., Camilleri, L., Bartolo, P., Grazzani, I., Cavioni, V., Conte, E., ... Colomeischi, A. (2022). The effectiveness of a school-based, universal mental health programme in six European countries. *Frontiers in Psychology, 8*(13), 925614. <https://doi.org/10.3389/fpsyg.2022.925614>.

Cefai, C., & Cavioni, V. (2014). *Social and emotional education in primary school: Integrating theory and research into practice.* Springer.

Cefai, C., Cavioni, V., Bartolo, B., Simões, C., Ridicki Miljevic, R., Bouillet, D., ... Eriksson, C. (2015). Social inclusion and social justice: A resilience curriculum for early years and elementary schools in Europe. *Journal of Multicultural Education, 9*(3), 122–139. <http://dx.doi.org/10.1108/JME-01-2015-0002>.

Cefai, C., & Cooper, P. (2009). *Promoting emotional education: Engaging children and young people with social, emotional and behavioural difficulties.* Jessica Kingsley Publishers.

Cefai, C., Ferrario, E., Cavioni, V., Carter A., & Grech, T. (2013). Circle time for social and emotional learning in primary school. *Pastoral Care in Education: An International Journal of Personal, Social and Emotional Development, 32*(2), 116–130.

Conte, E., Cavioni, V., Ornaghi, V., Agliati, A., Gandellini, S., Frade Santos., M., ... Grazzani, I. (2023). Supporting preschoolers' mental health and academic learning through the PROMEHS program: A training study. *Children, 10*(6), 1070.

Cooper, P. (2011). Teacher strategies for effective intervention with students presenting social, emotional and behavioural difficulties: An international review. *European Journal of Special Needs Education, 26*(1), 71–86.

Cooper, P. (2017). Building social-emotional resilience in schools. *Education in the Asia-Pacific Region, 28*, 489–506.

Cooper, P., & Cefai, C. (2013). Evidence-based approaches to social, emotional and behavior difficulties in schools. *KEDI Journal of Educational Policy, 10*(3), 81–101.

Cooper, P., & McIntyre, D. (1996). *Effective teaching and learning: Teachers' and students' perspectives.* Open University Press.

Cooper, P., & Tiknaz, Y. (2007). *Nurture groups in school and at home: Connecting with children with social, emotional and behavioural difficulties.* Jessica Kingsley Publishers.

Dickenson, P., Keough, P., & Courduff, J. (2016). *Preparing pre-service teachers for the inclusive classroom.* IGI Global.

Dunne, C. M. (2019). Primary teachers' experiences in preparing to teach Irish: Views on promoting the language and language proficiency. *Studies in Self-Access Learning Journal, 10*(1), 21–43.

European Agency for Development in Special Needs Education. (2012). *Teacher education for inclusion: Project recommendation linked to sources of evidence.* EADSNE.

Fredrickson, B. L., & Branigan, C. (2005). Positive emotions broaden the scope of attention and thought-action repertoires. *Cognition and Emotion, 19*(3), 313–332.

Grazzani, I., Agliati, I., Cavioni, V., Conte, E., Gandellini, G., Lupica Spagnolo, M., ... O'riordan, M. R. (2022). Adolescents' resilience during COVID-19 pandemic and its mediating role in the association between SEL and mental health. *Frontiers in Psychology, 7*(13), 801761.

Höltge, J., Jefferies, P., Cowden, R. G., Govender, K., Maximo, S. I., Carranza, J. S., ... Ungar, M. (2021). A cross-country network analysis of adolescent resilience. *Journal of Adolescent Health, 68*(3), 580–588.

Jennings, P. A., & Greenberg, M. T. (2009). The prosocial classroom: Teacher social and emotional competence in relation to student and classroom outcomes. *Review of Educational Research, 79*(1), 491–525.

Kane, R., Sandretto, S., & Heath, C. (2002). Telling half the story: A critical review of research on the teaching beliefs and practices of university academics. *Review of Educational Research, 72*(2), 177–228.

Lester, L., Cefai, C., Cavioni, V., Cross, D., & Barnes, A. (2020). A whole-school approach to promoting staff wellbeing. *Australian Journal of Teacher Education, 45*(2). <http://dx.doi.org/10.14221/ajte.2020v45n2.1>.

Limone, P., & Toto, G. A. (2022). Psychological strategies and protocols for promoting school well-being: A systematic review. *Frontiers in Psychology, 13*, 914063.

Mahoney, J. L., Weissberg, R. P., Greenberg, M. T., Dusenbury, L., Jagers, R. J., Niemi, K., ... Yoder, N. (2021). Systemic social and emotional learning: Promoting educational success for all preschool to high school students. *American Psychologist, 76*(7), 1128–1142.

Martinsone, B., Stokenberga, I., Damberga, I., Supe, I., Simões, C., Lebre, P., ... Camilleri, L. (2022). Adolescent social emotional skills, resilience and behavioral problems during the COVID-19 pandemic: A longitudinal study in three European countries. *Frontiers in Psychiatry, 13*, 942692.

Murray, C., & Pianta, R. C. (2007). The importance of teacher-student relationships for adolescents with high incidence disabilities. *Theory into Practice, 46*(2), 105–112.

Nalipay, M. J. N., King, R. B., Haw, J. Y., Mordeno, I. G., & Dela Rosa, E. D. (2021). Teachers who believe that emotions are changeable are more positive and engaged: The role of emotion mindset among in- and preservice teachers. *Learning and Individual Differences, 92*, 102050.

O'Connor, E. E., Dearing, E., & Collins, B. A. (2011). Teacher-child relationship and behavior problem trajectories in elementary school. *American Educational Research Journal, 48*(1), 120–162.

Richardson, V. (1996). The role of attitudes and beliefs in learning to teach. In J. Sikula (Ed.), *Handbook of research on teacher education* (pp. 102–119). Macmillan.

Saloviita, T. (2020). Attitudes of teachers towards inclusive education in Finland. *Scandinavian Journal of Educational Research, 64*(2), 270–282.

Toto, G. A. (2021). *Percezioni di efficacia e sviluppo professionale dei docenti*. Progedit.

Toto, G. A., & Limone, P. (2021). Motivation, stress and impact of online teaching on Italian teachers during COVID-19. *Computers, 10*, 75.

SU QIONG XU

7 The Curriculum Reforms of Special Education in the Context of Inclusive Education in China

Introduction

This chapter is inspired by Paul Cooper's idea of 'educational engagement' that emphasises all students' active participation in learning, though different provisions might need to be in place. This, to a certain extent, is similar to the Chinese government's action about improving educational equality for students with disabilities. This chapter thus discusses the curriculum reforms in special education in the context of the Chinese government's push toward inclusion. It first focuses on the historical development of special education curriculum reforms in China, and then discusses the challenges to further promote inclusive-oriented curriculum reforms in the dual-track education system of China. Finally, it makes several suggestions on the need for further curriculum reforms to ensure educational equity and quality for all.

Background

Inclusive education, as an ideological position of pursuing social justice and equality of access to education (Cooper & Jacobs, 2011), has resulted in worldwide education reforms to reconstruct schooling systems and provide appropriate aids for pupils with diverse learning needs in mainstream schools. As an initiative for inclusion in China, the *Learning in Regular Classrooms* (LRC) is a pragmatic strategy of the Chinese government to increase the school enrollment rate of school-aged children with disabilities (CWD). By 2020, around 49.47% (435,800) of CWD have been enrolled in mainstream schools to learn alongside their non-disabled peers (MOE, 2021). As a result, the LRC has contributed to not only improving access to compulsory education for the large population of CWD but also enhancing the quality of educational provision for them (Xu, Cooper & Sin, 2018).

The Chinese government is not only vigorously promoting inclusive education, but also providing separate special schools with trained professionals and specially designed resources (XU, Cooper & Sin, 2021). The LRC has become a crucial strategy to enhance the quality of educational provision for learners with disabilities, and the separate special schools are now evolving into resource centres to promote the inclusion of students with disabilities in mainstream classrooms. They are required to fully utilize their resources to promote inclusive practices in mainstream schools. Encountering multiple categories and various degree of disabilities, however, makes it difficult for the special schools to address individual needs effectively. It is also quite a challenge for them to operate as resource centres in relation to the education for all agenda posed by the dual-track education system in China.

From 1949 to today, the Chinese government has initiated five curriculum reforms for separate special schools and established a relatively complete curriculum framework and standards for special schools. This has not only greatly improved the quality of compulsory education for CWD in special schools, but also laid a foundation for inclusive-oriented curriculum reform in the future. This chapter thus aims to discuss curriculum reform in special education in the context of the Chinese government's push toward inclusion, by presenting curriculum reforms in the special education system, discussing the major challenges of inclusive-oriented curriculum reforms in the dual-track education system of China, and providing suggestions on how to promote inclusive education in China and countries like China.

The Curriculum Reforms of Special Education from 1949 to 2021

The Curriculum Reforms before the Market-oriented Reform (1949–1978)

At the beginning of the founding of the People's Republic of China, a highly centralised curriculum management mode was adopted, reflecting the former Soviet Union's educational theories and concepts such as *'teaching plan'* and *'textbook'*. To form a highly unified curriculum policy, the Chinese basic education system replaced *'curriculum theory'* with *'teaching theory'* and cancelled elective courses. The special education system was also influenced by the Soviet Union's educational theories and curriculum practices.

In 1957, the Chinese Education Committee (CEC) (renamed as the Ministry of Education in 1998, MoE) issued the *Instructions on Running Schools for Blind Children and Deaf-Mute Schools* to set basic requirements concerning the age of admission, class size, and teaching staff for the blind schools and the deaf-mute schools (Gu et al., 2010). In 1962, the CEC issued two programmatic documents: *The Six-year Full-time Teaching Plan for Blind Children (Draft)* and the *Ten-year Full-time Teaching Plan for Deaf-Mute Schools (Draft)* (Gu et al., 2010). The two drafts specified the development of objectives, teaching schedules, curriculum arrangements, and implementation of teaching plans for the blind and the deaf-mute schools. The basic task of the two types of special schools was to ensure that the blind, and the deaf and mute students have cultural and scientific knowledge, professional labour skills, and moral qualities as citizens. It is worth noting that the term *'deaf'* and *'mute'* always appear together in government documents, implying a common perception that those who are deaf are also mute. This reflects the lack of understanding of disability at that time. The teaching programmes and content of the blind and the deaf-mute schools were mainly taken from those of the general schools. These policy documents were the first special education curriculum reforms in China and laid the foundations for future curriculum reforms in the special education system of China. However, during *the Cultural*

Revolution (1966–1976), the development of special education in China was in a state of suspension, and many special schools were closed or disbanded.

The Local Exploration (1979–2000)

After the market-oriented reform in 1979, Chinese special education was gradually restored and rebuilt. In 1984, the CEC issued the *Teaching Plan for Full-time Deaf-Mute Schools* that flexibly divided the original unified school system into eight-year and six-year teaching plans in accordance with the unbalanced development of different regions in China (He, 1998). In 1985, the CEC published the *Decision of the Central Committee of the Communist Party on Reforming the Education System* to 'develop special education for blind, deaf, mute, disabled and mentally retarded children' (MoE, 1985). It was the first time that education for the 'mentally retarded' was mentioned (Zhao, 2008). In 1987, the CEC further issued the *'Teaching Plan for Full-time Blind Schools (Draft)'*, and the *'Teaching Plan for Full-time Mentally Retarded Schools (Class) (Draft)'* (He, 1998).

The above three teaching programmes signified the second special education curriculum reform in China. They build on the curriculum framework of the two Drafts of 1962, focusing on the responsibility of the three types of special schools to promote students' comprehensive development according to the principle of deficit compensation. This suggests that the second special education curriculum reform started to consider the particularities of CWD. It did not only pioneer the education of intellectual disabilities but also promoted the concept of the LRC by placing CWD who were capable of learning academic subjects into general schools. Furthermore, a series of teaching materials on specific subjects such as Chinese, mathematics, ideology and morality course, and music, was published to promote curriculum practices according to the teaching plans for the deaf-mute and the blind schools.

Further exploration was initiated under the impetus of a series of legislation in the 1990s (e.g. *the Compulsory Education Law of 1986, the Law on the Protection of Persons with Disabilities of 1990, and the Education Regulations of Persons with Disabilities of 1994*). This constituted the third special education curriculum reform in China. In 1993, the MoE launched the *Curriculum Plan for Full-time Schools for the Deaf (Trial)* and the *Curriculum Plan for Full-time Schools for the Blind (Trial)* to customise nine-year compulsory education for the deaf and blind (He, 1998). The term '*deaf*' was adopted to replace the term '*deaf-dumb*', reflecting a clear understanding of the differences between the deaf and the mute children. Perhaps because of a limited understanding of the nature of intellectual disability in the 1990s, the MoE did not release a curriculum plan for full-time schools of this group. Instead, the MoE published textbooks for the schools for the mentally retarded and began to use these nationwide. Subsequently, the *Outline of Education and Training for Students with moderate mental retardation (Trial)* was released in 1994 (Huang et al., 2019). In 1996, a whole set of new teaching materials for the deaf also began to be used across the country, and the principle of '*one guideline, multiple textbooks*' was proposed for the management, distribution, and use of the teaching materials.

The third special education curriculum reform in China adopted the term '*curriculum plan*' to replace the '*teaching plan*' in the documents of the previous two reforms. The two curriculum plans, and one outline helped to unify the school system in the 1990s. Moreover, moral education was strengthened by adding ideology and morality education and political education in deaf schools. Meanwhile, the curriculum provision in both the deaf and blind schools was improved, for example, replacing music with rhythm in the deaf schools teaching and introducing orientation as a subject in the blind school. A major change in the third special education curriculum reform of China was related to expanding the curriculum autonomy of the local education departments and schools, including the special schools. Along with such major changes in curriculum management, some schools also began to explore school-based curricula, and many school-based textbooks with local or school own characteristics were published across the country.

The Formation of Modern Curriculum System of Special Education in China (2001 until Now)

In 2001, the Chinese government initiated the basic education curriculum reform that emphasised the idea of *'paying attention to the development of every student'* (Zhong, 2021). This coincides with the concept of inclusive education that aims at education for all. It was realised that the basic education curriculum reform provided a great opportunity for inclusive-oriented curriculum developments. In 2003, the MoE launched the fourth special education curriculum reform by inviting researchers and professionals to analyse both the domestic and foreign literature and to conduct field research, in order to establish a new curriculum scheme for the three types of special schools. In 2007, the MoE released the three *Experimental Curriculum Schemes* to further promote compulsory education for the blind, the deaf, and children with intellectual disabilities, respectively (MoE, 2007). The three *Experimental Curriculum Schemes* reconstructed curriculum frameworks of special schools according to the idea of potential development and deficit compensation, the characteristics of the three types of disabilities, and the requirement of compulsory education that attaches significance to educational fairness, balance, and unity. However, the three *Experimental Curriculum Schemes* were merely curricular frameworks without specific details in relation to what and how to deliver the curriculum in practice for the three types of disabilities. The special schools had to try to carry out school-based experimental practices by themselves. Many special schools for intellectual disabilities tried to conduct curricular reforms in relation to individual education plans (IEP). As a result, a substantial number of model special schools of curriculum reform sprung up across the country.

In 2016, the MoE further released the *Curriculum Standards* of Compulsory Education for the blind, the deaf, and the intellectual disability respectively, based on the three *Experimental Curriculum Schemes* of 2007 (MoE, 2016). The three Curriculum Standards are the first set of systematic learning standards, especially for CWD in the Chinese history of special education. Compared to the three *Experimental Curriculum Schemes* of 2007, the 2016 *Curriculum Standards* were more specific in terms of curriculum standards and teaching implementation, and more flexible in terms of curriculum practices, adding selective curriculum, and encouraging innovations of teaching models in special schools. Moreover, the three *Curriculum Standards* involved some specially designed curricula (e.g. the registration for the blind, communication for the deaf, and rehabilitation training for intellectual disabilities) that responded to the ideas of potential development and deficit compensation and promoted the holistic development of learners with disabilities. The new teaching materials and supporting teaching references, which were uniformly organised and compiled by the MoE, have been implemented nationwide.

The Challenges in Implementing Inclusive-Oriented Curriculum Reforms in the Dual-Track Education System in China

The Problems of Reforming a Curriculum Based on Disability Categories

At present, the Chinese government has established relatively complete curriculum frameworks and standards for the three types of special schools. However, the current curriculum frameworks and standards are inadequate to meet the educational needs of students with other types of disabilities and with severe disabilities. Moreover, around 23% of students with multiple and severe disabilities are educated at home (MoE, 2021). Home-bound schooling for such students is inadequate in terms of curriculum and teaching, and thus unable to guarantee educational quality (Yang & Zhao, 2018). Under these circumstances, questions arise about how to initiate curriculum reforms to consider the educational needs of children with other types of disabilities, multiple and severe disabilities. It is also problematic to establish curriculum and teaching systems for preschools, high schools, vocational schools, and higher education according to types of disabilities.

The Integration of the General Curriculum and Special Curriculum

Through the five curriculum reforms, the special education system has established a relatively comprehensive curriculum framework for special schools. The fifth special curriculum reform, not only highlights the fundamental characteristics of the curriculum in relation to accomplishing compulsory education for all children but it also illustrates governmental move toward inclusion (Xu et al., 2021). However, the practice and process of special education curriculum are still separated from general schools. As a parallel system, the general schools find it difficult to take care of CWD.

Curriculum Authority and Autonomy

The five curriculum reforms of special education have illustrated a change from highly centralised curriculum management to a certain degree of curriculum autonomy. According to the basic education curriculum reform in 2001, the MoE allocated 20% curriculum autonomy to local schools. The increasing diversity of students' disabilities in general schools and the moderate and severe degrees of disabilities in special schools called for a higher degree of curriculum autonomy. However, the MoE has been tightening curriculum autonomy since 2014 (Long & Yu, 2019). Under these circumstances, there is little room for curriculum autonomy, which is not conducive to catering for individual differences. Despite the new curriculum standards having some flexibility, the overall implementation still follows a top-down strategy. As a result, more than 70% of special schools have not made a complete plan to implement the new curriculum standards (Xu, Xu & Wang, 2020). This implies that schools and teachers lack initiative in practice, and the reform process in schools is very slow.

The Challenge of Curriculum Implementation

In a recent study, Xu, Xu and Wang (2020) reported that the three types of special schools in China have started to implement the national curriculum standards of 2016, including organising training for teachers, using new textbooks, and adjusting teaching practices according to national curriculum standards. However, the majority of the schools in the study have not figured out the core of the new curriculum standards. For example, despite the setup of subjects according to curriculum standards, their teaching practices still follow the traditional teaching model of general schools, without fundamental change.

Moreover, among 2,244 special schools in China (MoE, 2021), 1,182 special schools were newly established or reconstructed from 2008 to 2012 (MoE, 2013). These schools were mainly located in the middle and west of China, with a relatively poor economy. In these schools, the quality of teaching is relatively poor, and their implementation of new curriculum standards is questionable.

Furthermore, compared to the deaf and blind schools, curriculum reform for schools with intellectual disabilities has been lagging behind. Both the first and the second special education curriculum reforms failed to consider schools for intellectual disabilities. The third reform published a series of teaching materials for students with intellectual disabilities without a curriculum plan. Although the fourth and fifth reforms have completed the curriculum framework, established national curriculum standards, and provided teaching contents and suggestions, the majority schools for intellectual disabilities find it difficult to implement the national curriculum because of the large differences among children with intellectual disabilities, and the enrollment of other types of disabilities (e.g. autism and cerebral palsy). There are also problems in the compilation of common textbooks for schools for intellectual disabilities according to national curriculum standards.

Professional Development

Teachers' professional development in special schools in China has been a problem. The latest national data shows that the rate of special education teachers and CWD is around 1:13.3 (MoE, 2021). Moreover, the majority of teachers did not graduate from special education major, while some teachers only received short-term training in special education. Under these circumstances, it is understandable that most special schools often report difficulties in implementing teaching according to the new curriculum standards (Xu, Xu, & Wang, 2020). Despite the new curriculum standards and new textbooks being widely adopted in special schools, the poor professional level of the teachers is one of the main challenges in implementing the new curriculum standards.

Meanwhile, along with the governmental push toward inclusive education, the Chinese LRC has greatly contributed to increasing the enrollment rate of school aged CWD in compulsory education. However, the LRC has been criticised as having poor quality in terms of catering for CWD attending general schools. A major challenge is related to the teachers' lack of acceptance of CWD (Xu & Cooper, 2020). Moreover, most general teachers have not received systematic and/or continuous training on the education of children with disabilities, despite the MoE's investment in national or provincial teacher training programs (Xu et al., 2018). Teachers lack awareness and understanding of individual differences and thus are not quite clear about the learning needs of CWD (Xu & Cooper, 2020). Furthermore, there is a serious shortage of resource teachers. Although the 2017 *Regulation on Education for Persons with Disabilities* encourages the developed regions of China to recruit resource teachers in general schools, most of them are part-time, and also in charge of teaching subjects such as Chinese and mathematics. They cannot focus on providing professional support for both the students with disabilities and the other teachers who are challenged by such students in their schools.

Recommendations

Establishing common curriculum framework. The dual-track education systems with different curriculum standards between the general and the special schools have been a major challenge to facilitating inclusive practice and policy implementation in China. It is crucial to establish a common curriculum framework for all schools that emphasises common goals for typical students and those with disabilities. It is not enough to establish consistent development goals at different learning stages in the common curriculum framework. Further development should focus on a curriculum model that not only builds on inclusion principles but also espouses greater flexibility in planning a curriculum suited to the needs of those with learning difficulties. The specific indicators of the common curriculum should involve academic goals in different subject areas (like Mathematics, Chinese, etc.), the goals of developing skills specifically for children with learning disabilities permeating all aspects of the curriculum areas, and particular attention to personal, social and health education and citizenship. By doing so, a national adaptation of the curriculum framework for children with various learning difficulties could be articulated to assist curriculum development in general schools.

Developing curricula and teaching guides for children with disabilities of various categories and degrees. Based on a common curriculum framework, it would be necessary to develop curriculum guides that support the learning needs of CWD of various categories and degrees and to provide guidelines for teachers to take care of those students in different educational placements. The curriculum guides should focus on discussing the possible functional problems of learning of CWD with various categories and degrees, and further provide potential solutions and strategies to address these issues. Moreover, cross-learning teaching or activities guidelines should be developed to provide a more practical reference for teachers.

Promoting practices of individual education plan and development of school-based curriculum. The school-based curriculum not only embodies curriculum autonomy but also reflects the advantages and characteristics of a school. Under the premise of implementing a common curriculum, both the general and special schools should continue to develop school-based curricula according to the characteristics and needs of their districts and schools, to further ensure quality and fairness. The IEP is an important embodiment of ensuring educational equality for CWD. Despite the 2017 *Regulation on Education for Persons with Disabilities* mentioning IEP for the first time, there is no normative requirement for how to develop and implement IEP. The latest evaluation indicated a messy situation of IEP development and implementation for CWD (Xin & Cao, 2016). Clearly legislation needs to regulate IEP development and implementation to guide teachers' practices.

Defining the responsibilities of the three levels of curriculum administration. The highly centralised curriculum management in China has ensured general uniformity, orderliness, and effectiveness of curriculum practices in schools, which is beneficial to guarantee the quality of teaching. There is still a need to strengthen curriculum authority to drive general education reform to establish a common curriculum framework for all. In this sense, the drive to strengthen curriculum authority in recent years in China might be beneficial to promote the reform of general education towards inclusive education, at least for now. Meanwhile, it is also important to leave some room for curriculum autonomy in the highly centralized education system. For local governments and schools, it is usually difficult to have their say in curriculum autonomy, with local curriculum management usually not being in place. It is important to clarify the responsibilities of curriculum management for the three main bodies, including the state, the local governments, and the schools, with more autonomy for the latter two.

Strengthening teachers' education programmes. Of a total of 3,005 colleges and universities in China, around 78 of them offer specialist or undergraduate courses to train pre-service professionals in special education. This is far from meeting the needs of education, research, and practices for persons with disabilities. The quantity and quality of pre-service teachers can be improved by properly expanding the enrollment scale of special education majors in colleges and universities, and by optimising the curriculum training programmes. Moreover, few colleges and universities offer elective curricula in special education for pre-service teachers in other majors. The

MoE should encourage all pre-service teachers to obtain credits in relation to taking care of students with learning difficulties.

Furthermore, the MoE and local departments should strengthen the in-service teachers' training by increasing investment and making appropriate training plans. Both the MoE and local education departments should encourage schools to carry out teaching and research on catering for individual differences, accumulating typical experiences and lessons, and promoting innovative exploration in the implementation process of curriculum reforms. This relates also to how effective teaching for individual differences in general classrooms should be understood, promoted and implemented (Cooper & McIntyre, 1996).

Conclusion

While segregated special schools are closing and inclusive education is advocated all over the world, China is one of the few countries that has built many segregated special schools and constantly promoted curriculum reforms for special schools. Through vigorous development of segregated special education, the Chinese government has greatly enhanced the awareness of education equity for persons with disabilities. Along with the five curriculum reforms of special education, education quality for persons with disabilities and professional development for special teachers have been improved significantly. Within the current drive towards inclusion, the segregated special schools in China are evolving into resource centres for CWD, taking responsibility for promoting inclusive practices in general schools in their own districts. In other words, the segregated special schools turn out to be the foundations for promoting inclusive education in China, rather than obstacles, at least for now. Such a phenomenon is an opposite of the 'universalist inclusion' which is against the existence of segregated special schools, including the issue of labelling and stigmatisation (Cooper & Jacobs, 2011). Labelling and other issues related to special education may serve to initiate general education reforms to cater to individual differences and to further establish an inclusive-oriented curriculum system in China.

References

Cooper, P., & Jacobs, B. (2011). *From inclusion to engagement: Helping students engage with schooling through policy and practices.* John Wiley & Sons.

Cooper, P., & McIntyre, D. (1996). *Effective teaching and learning: Teachers' and students' perspectives.* Open University Press.

Gu, D., Piao, Y., & Liu, Y. (2010). *Zhongguo teshu jiaoyushi ziliaoxuan (volume 2) [Historical resource of special education in China]* (pp. 1560–1621). Beijing Normal University Publication.

He, C. (1998). *Zhonghua renmin gongheguo zhongyao jiaoyu wenxian [Cruial references of education in the People's Republic of China]* (pp. 107–3565). Hainan Publication.

Huang, Z., Zeng, F., & Liu, C. (2019). Xinzhongguo chengli 70nianlai woguo teshu jiaoyu kecheng gaige de huigu yu qianzhan [70 years of curriculum reform in special education: review and prospect]. *The Chinese Journal of Special Education, 2019*(12), 3–11.

Long, A., & Yu, W. (2019). The reform and development of the basic education curriculum in China over the past 70 years. *The Journal of Curriculum, Teaching Material and Method, 39*(2), 11–18.

Ministry of Education (MoE). (1985). *Jiaoyu tizhi gaige wenxian xuanbian [A source book of reform on education system]* (p. 7). Education Science Publication.

Ministry of Education. (2007). *The notice of releasing "Experimental curriculum schemes of compulsory education for blind schools, deaf schools and intellectual disabilities schools".* Retrieved from <http://www.moe.gov.cn/srcsite/A06/s3331/200702/t20070202_128271.html>.

Ministry of Education. (2013). *Summary of special education development in China.* Accessed 19 January 2022. <http://www.moe.gov.cn/jyb_xwfb/s5147/201307/t20130715_154169.html>.

Ministry of Education. (2016). *The notice of implementing "Curriculum standards of compulsory education for the blind" "Curriculum standards of compulsory education for the deaf" "Curriculum standards of compulsory education for the intellectual disability".* Retrieved from <http://www.moe.gov.cn/srcsite/A06/s3331/201612/t20161213_291722.html>

Ministry of Education. (2021). *2020 nian quanguo jiaoyu shiye fazhan tongji gongbao. [Basic statistics of special education]*. Retrieved from 2020. <http://www.moe.gov.cn/jyb_sjzl/sjzl_fztjgb/202108/t20210827_555004.html>. (In Chinese).

Xin, W., & Cao, S. (2016). IEP making, implementation and challenge in the schools of intellectual disabilities: An investigation based on Hangzhou. *The Chinese Journal of Special Education, 2016*(4), 1–9.

Xu, S. Q., & Cooper, P. (2020). Mainstream teachers' perceptions of individual differences among students in inclusive education settings of China. *International Journal of Inclusive Education*. <https://doi.org/10.1080/13603116.2020.1735541>.

Xu, S. Q., Cooper, P., & Sin, K. (2018). The 'Learning in Regular Classrooms' initiative for inclusive education in China. *International Journal of Inclusive Education, 22*(1), 54–73.

Xu, S. Q., Cooper, P., & Sin, K. (2021). From inclusive-oriented curriculum to inclusive pedagogy: The realization of inclusion education. *Hong Kong Journal of Special Education, 22*, 55–65.

Xu, Z., Xu, S., & Wang, Y. (2020). Analysis and suggestions on the implementation of the new curriculum standards in special education school. *The Chinese Journal of Special Education, 2020*(9), 22–28.

Yang, S., & Zhao, B. (2018) Connotation, dilemma and suggestions on 'Homebound Instruction'. *The Journal of Suihua University, 38*(10), 20–23.

Zhao, X. (2008). Gaige kaifang 30nian zhongguo teshu jiaoyu de fazhan ji zhengce jianyi [Development and policy suggestions for Special education after 30 years' open-up reform in China]. *The Chinese Journal of Special Education*, (10), 35–41.

Zhong, Q. (2021). Cong zhishibenwei zhuanxiang suyangbenwei: kecheng gaige de tiaozhanxing keti [The challenge issue from knowledge-based to literacy-based curriculum reform]. *The Chinese Journal of Basic Education Curriculum*, (11), 5–20.

PART III

Nurture Groups

DAVID COLLEY

8 From Nurture Groups to Nurturing Cities: The Impact of Evidence-Based Research

Introduction

This chapter provides a critical analysis of the impact of Paul Cooper's research into nurture groups and nurturing schools. Nurture groups are a form of educational provision for children with social, emotional, behavioural and learning difficulties. Established by practitioners in the 1970s, it was the seminal research led by Cooper and colleagues that provided hard evidence for the success and worth of nurture group intervention. In Scotland, the six principles of nurture have been embraced by the city of Glasgow and the move towards 'the nurturing city' is well underway. In this chapter the influence of Cooper's work in providing the foundations for Glasgow's innovative approach is critically evaluated.

The Emergence of Nurture Groups in the UK

A nurture group is a form of educational provision that supports the social, emotional and mental health needs of children and young people (CYP) struggling to function constructively in the mainstream classroom environment (Colley & Seymour, 2021). Through the lens of nurture, troubling behaviours in school are understood to be a communication of an unmet need and the nurture group offers a safe base where carefully planned routines promote an increased sense of security and self-worth (Reynolds et al., 2009).

The 'classic' nurture group (Cooper & Whitebread, 2007) offers a routinised and predictable learning environment (Cooper & Tiknaz, 2007) that is well-led and well-taught (Ofsted, 2011). The nurture group is staffed by two experienced professionals who have undertaken specific training in the *Theory and Practice of Nurture Groups* (nurtureuk, 2023) which includes the fundamentals of attachment theory (Bowlby, 1969, 1973, 1980), the six Principles of Nurture (Insley, Lucas & Buckland, 2006) and social-emotional assessments through the Boxall Profile (Bennathan & Boxall, 1998). Nurture groups are designed to offer a small group of 10–12 CYP a safe base where group activities focus on addressing unmet social-emotional needs. Well-paced social activities, schemes of learning and the nurture breakfast all offer the opportunity for CYP to revisit early learning experiences that they may have missed (Boxall, 2002). Relationships and mutual trust are at the core of nurture group practice and staff will attune to the needs of CYP and co-regulate emotional outbursts with warmth, care and understanding (Colley, 2012).

The nurture team will identify and specify the CYP's unmet needs using the Boxall Profile assessment instrument and plan appropriate activities that allow social skills to be developed and enhanced. Following a part time placement in the nurture group, CYP will return to a full-time mainstream placement with a range of enhanced social-emotional skills. Evidence suggests that these improved skills can include 'improved concentration, behaviour and ability to learn' (Ofsted, 2005, p. 14), improved relationships with adults (DfES, 2005), enhanced emotional skills in the secondary school context (Colley, 2012; Chiappella, 2015) and statistically significant improvements in school functioning (Cloran et al., 2022).

The development of nurture groups and nurturing practices in schools began in London in the early 1970s through the innovative work of Marjorie Boxall (2002) and colleagues including Sylvia Lucas (1999, 2010, 2015). Although interest in nurture groups declined for a period in the 1980s, nurture group practice re-emerged in the 1990s thanks to the energy of Marion Bennathan (1996) – who led the original *Nurture Group Consortium* that is now *nurtureuk* – and the research evidence on nurture groups presented by Paul Cooper and colleagues between 1999 and 2017 (see Cooper et al.,

1999, 2001; Cooper, 2002, 2004a, 2006, 2010a, 2011; Cooper & Tiknaz, 2007, 2009; Colley & Cooper, 2017).

Cooper's extensive research interests and scholarship invariably has a focus on the wellbeing of children and young people and include seminal publications on ADHD (Cooper, 1997, 2008a; Gwernan-Jones, Cooper et al., 2016), attachment (Cooper, 2008b; Colley & Cooper, 2017) and the biopsychosocial model of social-emotional functioning (Upton & Cooper, 1990; Cooper, 1997; Cooper & Upton, 2006b; Cooper & Whitebread, 2007). But Cooper's interest in nurture groups as a practical and effective means of supporting emotional and behavioural difficulties has been a recurring theme throughout his research career and his publications have laid the foundations for innovative, evidence-based practice at home and abroad (see Cooper et al., 1999, 2001; Cooper, 2002, 2004a, 2006; Cooper & Tiknaz, 2007, 2009; Cooper 2010a, 2011; Colley & Cooper, 2017).

An Evidence-Based and Innovative Approach to Nurture Groups: The Scottish Experience

The influence of Cooper's research, scholarship and professional collaborations can be linked with many of these national and international developments through research citations and the development of his research themes. But this influence is particularly evident in Scotland where Cooper's work has been cited in large scale nurture group research projects (Reynolds et al., 2009), discussions around the future direction for nurture in education (Mackay, 2015) and the development of 'whole establishment nurturing projects' in Scotland (Kearney & Nowek, 2017).

In 1999, Cooper and colleagues published the first influential research paper to consider the nature and distribution of nurture groups in England and Wales (Cooper, Arnold & Boyd, 1999). This paper identified the key characteristics by which a genuine nurture group could be defined while also articulating four basic variations of the nurture group theme. The key nurture group characteristics that were articulated by the paper included an understanding of the developmental needs of children – and this became the first of six nurture principles that were to be set out in 2006 (Insley et al., 2006) and that continue to shape nurture group practice in Scotland (Figure 8.1). The paper also offered early warnings about nurture group variants that might contravene, undermine, or distort the key defining principles of the 'classic' nurture group and become 'sin bins' for children and young people.

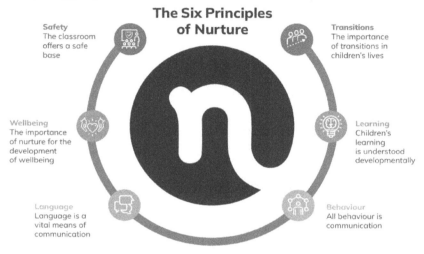

Figure 8.1. The Six Principles of Nurture (courtesy of nurtureuk)

Following their initial paper, Cooper, Arnold and Boyd (2001) then published the preliminary findings on the effectiveness of nurture groups that found clear evidence from interviews with teachers that nurture groups were perceived to have a positive influence on schools as a whole. For example, it was found that more nurturing attitudes and practices developed throughout the school and that changes in the ways in which teachers thought and talked about children were evident. Parents were consulted by the researchers and the majority of parents felt that placement in the nurture group had had a positive effect on the social, emotional and behavioural development of their children.

It should be noted that during this period, Cooper worked closely with Marion Bennathan and the emerging Nurture Group Consortium in developing the *Theory and Practice of Nurture Group* training that informs the current nurture training delivered in Scotland by the Psychological Services (Glasgow PS, 2023).

Cooper's collaborative work with Yonca Tiknaz provided more clear evidence regarding the impact of nurture group practice. Their paper *Progress and challenge in Nurture Groups: Evidence from three case studies* (Cooper & Tiknaz, 2005) identified ways in which nurture group practice could become a more coherent and sustained intervention. While the research identified communication between nurture staff and mainstream colleagues as a weakness across three case studies, attending the nurture group was seen to promote pupil progress in social-emotional functioning and this was confirmed by both nurture staff and mainstream staff. An additional area developed by this paper was the idea of creating 'a nurturing school' given the finding that a nurture group on site influenced mainstream culture and practice. The development of the nurturing school, first mooted by Lucas (1999) and Doyle (2003) has since been embraced by Education Scotland (2017), nurtureuk (National Nurturing Schools Training, 2023) and innovative current research projects (e.g. Colley & Seymour, 2023).

The final Cooper research paper to be cited in the Scottish innovations around nurture was published in 2007 with a focus on establishing the effectiveness of nurture groups on student progress and the impact of nurture groups on whole schools (Cooper & Whitebread, 2007). In this national research study, Cooper and Whitebread set out to measure (1) the effects of Nurture Groups in promoting pupil improvement in the Nurture Groups; (2) the extent to which these improvements generalised to mainstream settings; and (3) the impact of Nurture Groups on whole schools. A total of 546 CYP participated across 34 schools and eleven Local Education Authorities in the UK. The research compared schools that hosted nurture groups with those that did not and also looked at the performance of mainstream pupils both with and without social-emotional difficulties.

The results were compelling. Statistically significant improvements were found for nurture group pupils in terms of their social, emotional and behavioural functioning and the greatest improvements were found to take place over the first two terms of the nurture placement. The large-scale research found good evidence to suggest that successful nurture groups contribute to the development of the 'nurturing school' and that schools with nurture groups tended to manage the social and emotional difficulties of mainstream pupils more effectively.

From Nurturing Groups to Nurturing Cities

It was following the publication of this important paper (Cooper & Whitebread, 2007) that a Scottish research team led by Reynolds, MacKay and Kearney, undertook a large scale, controlled study of the effects of nurture group intervention on development and academic attainment across thirty-two schools in the City of Glasgow, Scotland (Reynolds et al., 2009). The measures central to this project included the Boxall Profile (Bennathan & Boxall, 1998), the Behavioural Indicators of Self Esteem (Burnett, 1998) and the Strengths and Difficulties Questionnaire (Goodman, 1997). On the Boxall Profile assessment, significant benefits were found for the nurture groups in comparison with the controls on all five Boxall Profile cluster areas, with significance levels ranging from $p = 0.003$ to $p < 0.001$. On the Behavioural Indicators of Self-esteem measure, significant benefits were found for the nurture groups v. controls ($p = 0.001$) although scores on the Strengths and Difficulties Questionnaire did not reach significant levels.

Following the publication of the positive results confirmed by Reynolds et al. (2009) in Glasgow, additional research was undertaken in Scotland around nurture group practice (e.g. MacKay, 2015; Fraser-Smith & Henry, 2016; Burns, MacDonald & Ferguson, 2018; Kearney & Nowek, 2019; Kearney et al., 2020; Carleton et al., 2021).

A clear programme around nurturing schools, nurturing communities and nurturing cities was also advanced in the policy document *Getting it Right in Glasgow, the Nurturing City* (Glasgow City Council, 2016). The stated aim of this pioneering policy was 'to guide and support progress in developing nurturing schools in a nurturing city' because it was Glasgow's ambition to become "the nurturing city"' (p. 3). Building on the principles of nurture that were developed through the research of Cooper, Lucas and others, the policy argues that a 'nurturing city' has schools in which 'children and young people feel they belong, they are listened to and (that) they and their families are valued'. In addition, the nurturing city seeks to ensure that 'all our children and young people will grow and learn in environments where they are safe and healthy, active, nurtured and achieving, respected, responsible and included. They will be valued as individuals and their needs will be understood and met' (p. 3).

Alongside the *Getting it right in Glasgow* policy document (2016), Education Scotland published the *Applying Nurture as a While School Approach Framework* (2017) which set out to support the self-evaluation of nurturing approaches in schools and early learning settings. In the Framework, the rationale for nurturing approaches emphasises the need to focus on well-being, relationships and the growth and development of children and young people. The six Principles of Nurture, developed through the work of Cooper et al. (2001), Boxall (2002) and Lucas et al. (2006) are included verbatim in the Framework while the nurturing approach 'recognises that positive relationships are central to both learning and wellbeing' (Education Scotland, 2017, p. 13).

In many respects, the Framework (Education Scotland, 2017) is at the cutting edge of nurturing approaches across schools and communities. It includes a self-evaluation process for schools and a detailed set of quality indicators around *How Nurturing is our Leadership? How Nurturing is the quality of care and education we offer? and How Nurturing are we in our approach?* Also included are Readiness Checklists (whole school nurture and individual nurture) and an Observation Profile that looks at the whole classroom environment and its explicit relationship to the six Principles of Nurture (Lucas et al., 2006). For example, are there clear routines visible in the classroom? Have safe spaces been created for CYP that might be overwhelmed at times by the mainstream classroom? Do staff use the language of co-regulation in crisis situations?

In addition, the Framework (Education Scotland, 2017) includes an Attunement Profile that helps practitioners to reflect on their own attunement styles based on Key Attuned Principles (e.g. encouraging and receiving initiatives in class, naming differences or contradictions, having fun and showing enjoyment). It is important to note that areas of development that staff identify for themselves regarding their own attunement skills are owned by the staff members and not peers or management. The Attunement Profile is about high-quality professional reflection, professional development and the embedding of nurturing principles into every crevice of school practice.

A Career Long Commitment to Nurture

Cooper (2010b) argued that the prevalence of children and young people with social, emotional and behavioural difficulties was, to a significant degree, a reflection of a maladjusted culture and that 'societies beget the children that they deserve' (Cooper, 2010, p. 7). Scotland is striving towards a well-adjusted culture – no matter how daunting that may be – in the hope that a move from nurture groups to nurturing cities may yet lead to 'a continuum of nurture to resolve the world's problems' (Lucas, 2019). Cooper's research and research collaborations, his inspiration to PhD students, his encouragement of co-authors and his career-long commitment to thinking about how best to support children with emotional difficulties have been the foundations upon which whole school nurturing practices have since flourished.

References

Bennathan, M., & Boxall, M. (1996). *Effective intervention in primary schools*. David Fulton Publishers.
Bennathan, M., & Boxall, M. (1998). *The Boxall profile: A guide to effective intervention in the education of pupils with emotional and behavioural difficulties*. Association of Workers for Children with Emotional and Behavioural Difficulties.
Boxall, M. (2002). *Nurture groups in school: Principles and practice*. Paul Chapman.
Bowlby, J. (1969). *Attachment and loss: Volume I attachment*. The Hogarth Press.

Bowlby, J. (1973). *Attachment and loss: Volume II separation anxiety and anger*. The Hogarth Press.
Bowlby, J. (1980). *Attachment and loss: Volume III sadness and depression*. The Hogarth Press.
Burnett, P. C. (1998). Measuring behavioural indicators of self-esteem in the classroom. *The Journal of Humanistic Education and Development, 37*, 107–116.
Burns, J., MacDonald, A., & Ferguson, N. (2018). Improving pupils' perceptions of the learning environment through enhanced nurturing approaches: An evaluation. *The International Journal of Nurture in Education, 4*(1), 33–44.
Carleton, R., Nolan, A., Murray, C., & Menary, S. (2021). Renfrewshire's nurturing relationships approach: Utilising nurturing approaches to support school staff and pupils during Covid-19. *The International Journal of Nurture in Education, 7*(1), 73–84.
Cefai, C., & Cooper, P. (2011). Nurture groups in Maltese schools: Promoting inclusive education. *British Journal of Special Education, 38*, 65–72.
Chiappella, J. (2015). Part-time secondary school nurture groups. *The International Journal of Nurture in Education, 1*(1), 15–24.
Cloran, P., Rivard, M., & Bennett, A. (2022). Classroom as a secure base and safe haven: Nurture group implementation in two Montreal schools. *The International Journal of Nurture in Education, 8*(1), 7–22.
Colley, D. (2009). Nurture groups in secondary schools. *Emotional and Behavioural Difficulties, 14*(4), 291–300.
Colley, D. (2012). *The development of nurture groups in secondary schools* [Thesis, University of Leicester]. Retrieved from <https://hdl.handle.net/2381/10132>.
Colley, D., & Cooper, P. (2017). *Attachment and emotional development in the classroom*. Jessica Kingsley Publishing.
Colley, D., & Seymour, R. (2021). An evidence-based guide to opening a successful secondary school nurture group. *International Journal of Nurture in Education, 7*(1), 56–72.
Colley, D., & Seymour, R. (2023). *The Mulberry Bush nurturing schools project* [Unpublished].
Cooper, P. (1997). Biology, behaviour and education: ADHD and the bio-psychosocial perspective. *Educational and Child Psychology, 14*, 31–38.
Cooper, P. (2002). The effectiveness of nurture groups: Preliminary research findings. In J. Visser (Ed.), *Emotional and behavioural difficulties: Successful practice* (pp. 9–17). Qed.
Cooper, P. (2004a). Nurture groups: The research evidence. In J. Wearmouth, R. C. Richmond, & T. Glynn (Eds), *Addressing pupils' behaviour: Responses at district, school and individual levels* (pp. 176–196). David Fulton.

Cooper, P. (2004b). Learning from nurture groups. *Education 3–13, 32*(3), 59–72. <https://doi.org/10.1080/03004270485200341>.

Cooper, P. (2006). Nurture groups 1970–2003. In M. Carsch, Y. Tiknaz, P. Cooper, & R. Sage (Eds), *The handbook of social, emotional and behavioural difficulties* (pp. 101–111). Publisher.

Cooper, P. (2008a). Like alligators bobbing for poodles? A critical discussion of education, ADHD and the biopsychosocial perspective. *Journal of Philosophy of Education, 42*(3–4), 457–474. <https://doi.org/10.1111/j.1467-9752.2008.00657.x>.

Cooper, P. (2008b). Nurturing attachment to school: Contemporary perspectives on social, emotional and behavioural difficulties. *Pastoral Care in Education, 26*, 13–22. <https://doi.org/10.1080/02643940701848570>.

Cooper, P. (2010a). Nurture groups: An evaluation of the evidence. In C. Cefai & P. Cooper (Eds), *Promoting emotional education: Engaging children and young people with social, emotional and behavioural difficulties* (pp. 133–143). Jessica Kingsley.

Cooper, P. (2010b). Social, emotional and behavioural difficulties in young people: The challenge for policy makers. *International Journal of Emotional Education, 2*(1), 4–16.

Cooper, P. (2011). Educational and psychological interventions for promoting social-emotional competence in school students: Mental health and wellbeing. In R. H. Shute (Ed.), *Mental Health and Wellbeing. Educational Perspectives* (pp. 29–40). Shannon Research Press.

Cooper, P., Arnold, R., & Boyd, E. (1999). *The nature and distribution of NGs in England and Wales.* University of Cambridge School of Education.

Cooper, P., Arnold, R., & Boyd, E. (2001). The effectiveness of nurture groups: Preliminary research findings. *British Journal of Special Education, 28*, 160–166.

Cooper, P., & Tiknaz, Y. (2005). Progress and challenge in nurture groups: Evidence from three case studies. *British Journal of Special Education, 32*, 211–222.

Cooper, P., & Tiknaz, Y. (2007). *Nurture groups in school and at home: Connecting with children with social, emotional and behavioural difficulties.* Jessica Kingsley.

Cooper, P., & Tiknaz, Y. (2010). Nurture groups in school and at home. In C. Cefai & P. Cooper (Eds), *Nurture groups in primary schools: The Maltese experience* (pp. 123–44). Verlag.

Cooper, P., & Upton, G. (2006b). An ecosystemic approach to emotional and behavioural difficulties in schools. *Educational Psychology, 10*, 301–321. <https://doi.org/10.1080/0144341900100402>.

Cooper, P., & Whitebread, D. (2007). The effectiveness of nurture groups on student progress: Evidence from a national research study. *Emotional and Behavioural Difficulties*, *12*(3), 171–190. <https://doi.org/10.1080/13632750701489915>.

Couture, C., Lavoie, C., Begin, J., & Masse, L. (2017). The differentiated impact of Kangaroo Class programmes in Quebec primary schools: Examining behavioural improvements in relation to student characteristics in 'nurture and nurture groups'. *Emotional and Behavioural Difficulties Special Issue*, *22*, 185–187.

Department for Education and Skills (DfES). (2005). *Learning behaviour: The report of the practitioners' group on school behaviour and discipline*. The Stationery Office.

Doyle, R. (2003). Developing the nurturing school: Spreading nurture group principles and practices into mainstream classrooms. *Emotional and Behavioural Difficulties*, *8*(4), 252–266.

Education Gazette (New Zealand) Aotearoa. (2021). *Nurturing the future*. Education Gazette <https://gazette.education.govt.nz/articles/nurturing-the-future/>

Education Scotland. (2017). *Applying nurture as a whole school approach*. <https://education.gov.scot/improvement/Documents/inc55ApplyingNurturingApproaches120617.pdf>

Fraser-Smith, J., & Henry, K. (2016). A systemic evaluation of a nurture group in Scotland. *The International Journal of Nurture in Education*, *2*(1), 37–44.

Glasgow City Council. (2016). *Getting it right in Glasgow, the nurturing city*. <https://www.glasgow.gov.uk/CHttpHandler.ashx?id=32783&p=0>

Glasgow PS. (2023). *Nurture – Glasgow Educational Psychology Service*. <https://blogs.glowscotland.org.uk/glowblogs/glasgowpsychologicalservice/nurture/>

Goodman, R. (1997). The strengths and difficulties questionnaire: A research note. *Journal of Child Psychology and Psychiatry*, *38*, 581–586.

Gwernan-Jones, R., Moore, D., Cooper, P., Russell, A., Richardson, M., Rogers, M., … Garside, R. (2016). A systematic review and synthesis of qualitative research: The influence of school context on symptoms of attention deficit hyperactivity disorder. *Emotional and Behavioural Difficulties*, *21*, 1–18.

Hughes, N., & Schlösser, A. (2014). The effectiveness of nurture groups: A systematic review. *Emotional and Behavioural Difficulties*, *19*(4), 386–409.

Kearney, M., & Nowel, G. (2019). Beyond nurture groups to nurturing approaches: A focus on the development of nurture in the Scottish context. *The International Journal of Nurture in Education*, *5*(1), 12–20.

Kearney, M., Crawford, A., Jennings, C., & Kerr, J. (2020). The nurturing establishment: Gathering children and parental/carer views of their experiences of a nurturing establishment. *The International Journal of Nurture in Education*, *6*(1), 13–24.

Lucas, S. (1999). The nurturing school. *Emotional and Behavioural Difficulties*, *4*(3), 14–19.

Lucas, S. (2010). *Nurture groups in schools* (2nd edn) (Boxall, M. 2002 rev.) Sage.

Lucas, S. (2019). On the origins of nurture. *International Journal of Nurture in Education*, *5*(1), 7–11.

Lucas, S., Insley, K., & Buckland, G. (2006). *Nurture group principles and curriculum guidelines: Helping children to achieve.* Nurture Group Network.

MacKay, T. (2015). Future directions for nurture in education: Developing a model and a research agenda. *The International Journal of Nurture in Education*, *1*(1), 33–40.

Nurtureuk. (2023). *Training and events.* Retrieved from <https://www.nurtureuk.org/what-we-do/training-and-events/>

Ofsted. (2005). *Managing challenging behaviour.* Ofsted.

Ofsted. (2011). *Supporting children with challenging behaviour through a nurture group approach.* <www.ofsted.gov.uk/resources/supporting-children-challenging-behaviour-through-nurture-group-approach>

Pace, M. (2022). Characteristics and experiences of nurture group and learning support zone educators in Malta. *The International Journal of Nurture In Education*, *8*, 37–47.

Reynolds, S., MacKay, T., & Kearney, M. (2009). Nurture groups: A large-scale, controlled study of effects on development and academic attainment. *British Journal of Special Education*, *36*(4), 204–212.

Sloan, S., Winter, K., Connolly, P., & Gildea, A. (2020). The effectiveness of nurture groups in improving outcomes for young children with social, emotional and behavioural difficulties in primary schools: An evaluation of nurture group provision in Northern Ireland. *Children and Youth Services Review*, *108*, 104619.

Upton, G., & Cooper, P. (1990). A new perspective on behaviour problems in schools: The ecosystemic approach. *Maladjustment & Therapeutic Education*, *8*, 3–18.

Welsh Assembly. (2010). *Nurture groups: A handbook for schools.* Cymry Ifanc.

CARMEL BORG

9 Returning from Educational Exile: The School of Barbiana and Emancipatory Nurture Groups as Projects of Hope and Possibility

Introduction

Together with fellow travellers, Paul Cooper dedicated substantial time and academic energy to explore the perennial challenge of how schools can re/engage alienated children by 'reattaching' them to transformative educational sites – schools or other educational spaces that operate differently from the unhospitable scholastic spaces which would have pushed children out (Cooper, 2008). While focusing on educational terrains, which can domesticate as much as they can emancipate, this chapter builds on the awareness that the highly demanding task of attracting children back to the educational realm – physically, mentally and emotionally – is often complicated by layers of injustices unfolding outside the periphery of the schooling system. It seeks to do so by examining how the School of Barbiana in Italy operated as an emancipatory, nurturing project fostering hope and possibility for its students.

Background

Education, while potentially liberating, has its limits. Asymmetrical access to education is symptomatic of unequal social relations beyond education, as the pandemic has unmistakably revealed (Borg, 2022a). In fact, life during Covid-19 mirrored the pre-pandemic material relations that have defined the power dynamics within neoliberalism's sphere of influence. The structurally informed difficulties experienced by families during the pandemic, partially induced by long years of the neoliberal state's withdrawal from an increasingly divisive social life, resulted in differentiated levels of educational participation and access for children (Borg, 2022b). Nurturing in education, a central theme in Cooper's academic and professional output, cannot ignore such asymmetries, as will be emphasised in this chapter.

In an age where individualism and self-servitude are elevated to hegemonic status, and where public goods continue to transition into the private realm, Emancipatory Nurturing in Education (ENiE) is hereby conceived of as a moment of resistance to expert-driven, unidirectional and deficit-oriented approaches to 'rehabilitating' or 'fixing' what is perceived as the broken child. Built on reciprocity and mutuality, and with the child and their significant others regarded as authentic collaborators, ENiE reclaims collective solidarity and consciousness-building as pedagogy of hope and socio-emotional possibility.

In responding to a liberatory conception of nurturing in education, this chapter critically reflects on the story of a nurture group, conceived and executed in institutional 'exile', more than fifty years ago; a nurture group created in resistance to an education system that selectively failed working-class children who, back then, were quickly and regularly dispatched to work either in the factories that fuelled the Italian economic miracle or, seasonally, in the nearby fields. Geographically situated in Tuscany's Mugello region, the nurture group created by don

Lorenzo Milani (1923–1967) responded to the children's immediate and most relevant needs, not only of survival but also of permanent freedom.

The School of Barbiana is a case study of an emancipatory nurture group, set against a backdrop of structural inequity in education and beyond; created specifically to rapture a predictable educational script where working-class children came out of school academically challenged and emotionally distraught, thinking that the reproduction of their social status and economic predicament were inevitable, and that they were naturally programmed to living precariously.

Rather than creating an ephemeral pit-stop that would help children survive scholastically, Milani's nurture group nourished permanence by welding functional literacy with critical reading and action on the world. It promoted personal and social emancipation for the long haul, an inspirational educational story that could serve as a catalyst for a movement of emancipatory nurture groups that sets its remit beyond reintegration into education systems that fail children.

A Chance Beginning

Don Lorenzo Milani arrived at Barbiana, a tiny parish on the Northern slope of Mount Giovi, Italy, in December 1954. The Curia of Florence had originally decided to close the remote and almost deserted parish. However, the decision was reversed on purpose, to host the rebellious don Milani. The transfer to Barbiana, in fact, was meant to subdue the priest's uncompromising critique of the Italian establishment, political parties and his beloved Catholic Church included. He often accused the leadership of the aforementioned secular-clerical establishment of alienating their faithful, depriving them of a real presence in the world, democratic engagement and critical citizenship (Borg et al., 2009).

The time spent in Barbiana, prior to his untimely death in 1967, at the young age of 44 years, proved to be a most productive period of his life. It was a critical-pedagogical experience culminating in a book – *Lettera a una professoressa* (Letter to a Teacher) – written by a group of students who arrived at Milani's nurturing space from a schooling system that had pushed them out. 'Letter to a Teacher' is a written testament to what can be achieved in an emancipatory nurture group, when civically-courageous, intellectually-prepared, socially-committed, fearless and transformation-oriented educators denounce the concept of students as deficient-others to be fixed, partially or wholly, out-of-sight of the 'gifted' others, and announce nurturing as an education process with an emancipatory twist.

The *Lettera* constitutes an attempt by children who had passed through a process of psychological, emotional, academic, ideological, ethical and moral awakening to lay bare the nuts and bolts of an exclusionary educational machine that served the asymmetrical society rather than the genuine inclusion of all children.

In the most direct and communicable language possible, understandable to all, the students reflected on their lived experience to illustrate how the social, economic and cultural capital of Pierino, the fictitious character in the letter, who represented the privileged cohort of children, set him on a different educational trajectory than that of working-class Gianni, with school playing a decisive role in offering a seamless journey to Pierino while persuading Gianni that he is unteachable. The captivating, generally angry account of the children is understandable given the rude awakening that they were given by a curriculum of life that had included several moments of conscientisation for critical citizenship; a pedagogical process where learning to read the word led to reading the world.

Anticipating the more sophisticated, academic studies of the 'new sociology of education', the students at Barbiana gave a very insightful account of how schooling had reinforced social and economic distinction through a culturally-biased curriculum, short hours of schooling exacerbated by long holidays, and 'authoritarian' teachers who were generally convinced that school failure was directly proportionate to innate limitations.

The students' scathing analysis of their educational journey, nurtured through a process of conscientisation, led by an authoritative educator, was widened in scope through data collection from the National Office of Statistics in Rome which revealed a positive correlation between socio-economic status and educational achievement. Through statistical analysis, an incredible cognitive feat given where the students were coming from educationally, the student-authors were able to illustrate how working-class children were disproportionately represented in the category of children who were being shortchanged by an education system bent at reproducing the asymmetrical status quo.

'I Care' – A Nurture Group with a Transformative Ethos

In response to the language of critique, don Milani's nurture group evolved into an educational site with an ethos that viewed schooling as a gift, at the service of people (Simeone, 2009). Best captured in the motto inscribed on one of its walls – *I Care* – it provided a conscious antidote to a school that autocratically imposed an educational regime that reproduced social, economic and cultural segregation.

At Barbiana, individualism and competition were replaced by collectivity and solidarity, transforming the school's motto into inclusion in action. In the boys' words:

> The following year I was a teacher. That is, I was a teacher for three-and-a-half days a week ... If I made mistakes it did not matter much. It was a relief for the boys. We looked up things together. The hours passed serenely, without fear and without feelings of submission. (School of Barbiana, 2009, p. 37)

Barbiana's ethos nurtured a key principle of inclusion – schools should not fail students; 'Nobody was hopeless for schooling' (School of Barbiana, 2009, p. 35). In the eyes of the student authors, a school that sorts, classifies and labels constitutes a social entrapment that structurally relegates a disproportionate number of working-class students to segregationist programmes that are often informed by low expectations or in-class tracking disguised as mainstreaming. In the words of the student-authors (2009):

> At the elementari the State offered me a second-class school. Five classes in one school hall. One fifth of the school that I had a right to.

> It is the system used in America in order to create differences between whites and blacks. Worse schools for the poor from when they are young (School of Barbiana, 2009, p. 34).

Emancipatory nurture groups in the image of Barbiana, resist segregation and exclusion, both temporary and permanent, because 'it's better to be considered mad, rather than being a tool of racism.' (School of Barbiana, 2009, p. 43).

With social transformation as a core aspect of the Barbiana group's ethos, critical literacy, (along with functional literacy) was key to consciousness building. Being present in the world to critically engage with and act on it was an indispensable feature given the negative self-perception drummed into Milani's students by a mainstream school that had failed them academically and socially. Such consciousness building, resulting from critical reflection on the world that is, lays the foundation for personal and collective action for a world that can be. The shift in the students' consciousness is exemplified in the following quote from the Letter, one of several, where the student-authors argue that:

> Schools have only one problem. The children that they lose.
>
> Your "compulsory schooling" loses 462,000 every year by the wayside. At this point, the only ones who are incompetent about schooling are yourselves, as you lose them and do not go back to find them. Not us, as we meet them in the fields or in the factories and we know them closely. (School of Barbiana, 2009, p. 57)

In response to such shift in consciousness, the School of Barbiana set the goal of rehumanising students who have been dehumanised by a system that generally favoured privileged students over their underprivileged counterparts.

> Wanted: an honest goal. Wanted: a goal.
>
> It has to be an honest one. A great one. That it does not presuppose anything in the child except that he is human. That is, it has to suit both believers and atheists (School of Barbiana, 2009, p. 109).

A human-rights-informed goal which cannot be reached unless one realises that 'it's more honest to say that all children are born equal and if at a later stage they are not equal anymore, it's our fault and we must remedy this' (School of Barbiana, 2009, p. 79). A realisation that is comforted by one's 'wish to love' and by dedicating 'oneself to one's neighbour', 'understand others' and '... make oneself understood' (School of Barbiana, p. 109). Emancipatory nurture groups are schools of 'social service' (School of Barbiana, 2009, p. 125), genuine hospitality and compassion beyond borders.

A Nurture Group Where the Pedagogical Experience Is Content

The pedagogical experience at Barbiana reflected the ethos of the nurture group. Peer tutoring, one of the foremost pedagogical tools that turned the 'I Care' ethos into a lived experience, was possible because Milani fostered a spirit and mentality of collaboration among the students.

In response to a curricular experience committed to personal and social emancipation, language, an aspect of cultural capital that often determines social presence, inclusion and engagement, featured prominently in the nurturing process:

Sovereign. Because only language can render equal. Equal is he who can express himself and he who understands the idiom of others (School of Barbiana, 2009, p. 110).

At Barbiana, daily and lengthy reading sessions, mostly from newspapers, were consciously designed to improve the students' proficiency in the standard form of the Italian language, conceived of by Milani as the language of power. While validating the students' regional dialect, Milani considered command of the official language as a vehicle for active and democratic citizenship, an aspect of the curricular experience that cannot be compromised by nurture grouping.

Don Milani's obsession with critical literacy as an instrument of liberation, drew from his objective observation that those who could not read and critically engage with the newspaper, one of the dominant forms of news transportation and manufacture of consent at his time, were easily pushed to a life of subordination and indoctrination.

Such was Milani's high expectations and unconditional belief in the cognitive abilities of his students, a necessary attitudinal prerequisite for successful emancipatory nurture groups, that his daily functional-cum-critical literacy sessions included challenging texts that dealt with complex political issues such as India's Independence and South Africa's apartheid system.

Apart from the long hours of schooling, the learning community at Barbiana was prepared to slow down the pace not to leave anyone behind. Slowing down also meant resistance to the frenetic pace imposed by capitalist economic and social relations, a function of Western modernity, where speed and efficiency, linked to profit at all cost and accumulation of wealth, are conceived of as indispensable characteristics of a viable world economic order.

Compared to normal school hours at the time, the educational hours spent at Barbiana were long, and were meant to cover both the official curriculum, as dictated centrally, as well as the 'curriculum of life', as informed by the real and tangible needs of the students. Long hours made it possible for the learning community created at Barbiana to reclaim lost ground, following years of experiencing a curricular culture that rarely came close to understanding the real needs of the community, such as a curricular experience that was tolerant of curricular interruptions, gave attention to irrelevant details, was inordinately preoccupied with linguistic exceptions and was chronically plagued by limited time-on-task. Such curricular characteristics generally favour students from privileged backgrounds; students who are not as dependent on school life for scholastic success as their underprivileged counterparts generally are.

Confidence building was nurtured assiduously within Barbiana's learning community. Milani argued that in the context of Barbiana, shyness was mainly a function of social-class subordination reproduced by a school history that infallibly shunned the underprivileged children. In the eyes of Milani, shyness forced the community into a 'culture of silence' and chronic fatalism, a state of mind that barred them from active democratic citizenship:

> Shyness. Two years ago, when I was in the prima magistrale class, you used to intimidate me. After all, my shyness has accompanied me all throughout my life. When I was young, I did not use to raise my eyes from the ground. I used to flatten myself against walls not to be seen.

> At first, I thought it was a sickness of mine, or, at the very most, of my family. My mother is one of those people who feel intimidated even when looking at a telegram. My father observes and listens, but he does not speak. (School of Barbiana, 2009, p. 33)

For Milani, genuine democratic participation requires emotional strength as much as intellectual preparation. not only to be able to be present in the world, but also to face and speak truth to power. In response to the need for emotional formation, the curricular experience at Barbiana included several initiatives that targeted confidence building.

One such initiative was the *Conferenza del Venerdi* (Friday conference). All week, students were prepared for a Friday encounter with Milani's invitees. Learned speakers were often surprised by the quality of questions asked and the assertiveness expressed by the students. The *conferenza* was not simply an act of intellectual enrichment and exchange. It also provided a safe space where students could build their emotional resilience by executing their civic courage to discomfort, ask difficult questions, and problematise expert knowledge. The Friday conference was a laboratory in intellectual and emotional resilience in action.

Aware of the importance of cultural and social capital to confidence building, the curricular experience at Barbiana included the hosting of a number of young foreigners with whom Milani's students could interact in English, French and German. In addition, a number of students would be encouraged to spend some time abroad.

Apart from helping students to overcome shyness and build emotional resilience, the trips in question also helped in building the student's social capital, intercultural skills in particular. It was through such an experience that linguistic skills served as an instrument of social relations, real exchange, culture and negotiation (Toriello, 2008).

No Reading of the World without Writing the World

Milani-inspired emancipatory nurture groups promote 'powerful skills' One such skill that featured prominently in Barbiana's curriculum was collective writing. Like peer tutoring, mentioned earlier, collective writing was seen by Milani as an opportunity for students to experience communality first-hand.

Influenced by Mario Lodi (1922–2014), an Italian educator and writer, who in turn was inspired by the cooperative-education school of the French pedagogue, Célestin Freineit (1896–1966), Milani taught students how to organise their thoughts into individual cards, then into sections, place them in a sequence and name each section. Once the paragraphs are put into a sequence, the language is filtered of difficult words, long sentences, repetitions, and overloaded and ambiguous sentences. This was all done collectively and with a commitment for popular communicability.

Since it was writing with a popular-political purpose, Milani's instructions regarding writing were very specific:

> Have something important to say, and that it may be useful to everybody or to many. To know who you are writing to. To gather all that is necessary. To find a logical way of putting it in order. To eliminate any unnecessary word. To eliminate any word which we do not use while speaking. Not to set any limits of time. (School of Barbiana, 2009, p. 44)

For Milani, a committed educator, the word cannot afford to say nothing or to repeat the obvious.

The Strategic Importance of Transformative Educators

In chapter four of his often-quoted book, Freire (1997) describes the indispensable qualities of progressive (read transformative) educators; a chapter which can help educators aspiring to engage in an emancipatory agenda for nurture groups to understand the built-in characteristics of a professional working in an area that is primarily interested in reclaiming humanity and citizenship. The chapter in question should also help the reader understand better how it was possible for don Milani, almost single-handedly, with very limited resources, against the institutional grain, in a remote and quasi-deserted part of the country and working with children who were systematically and systemically being pushed out of the education system, to achieve results that overly-resourced and credentialed educators may not come close to achieving.

Humility (a function of self-confidence, self-respect and respect for others), lovingness, courage, tolerance, experience of the tension between patience and impatience, scientific competence, and joy of living are the qualities mentioned by Freire in the fourth letter to the teachers 'who dare teach'. Milani mirrored these qualities in: his *courage* to publicly confront the manufactured consent that working-class children were destined to fail, and in facing the ire of parents who initially resisted his educational project because they had fatalistically accepted that their children's predicament was part of their destiny; his militant and rebellious *love* for humanity, leaving a very comfortable life within an upper-middle-class family to live a life of austerity, serving the economically and socially disadvantaged sector of society, against a backdrop marked by a very hostile political and ecclesiastical environment, and a terminal illness that had eaten into his quality of life for ten years of his short life; his *patience,* spending long hours with the students, engaging reflectively with the world, and his *impatience* in acting on the world through intense public engagement, culminating in a book removed from the commercial book shelves in 1958, a court case for conscientiously objecting to universal conscription, and the 'Letter to a Teacher', published in 1967; his *humility* shown in his ability to listen to the real needs of the children and in creating a 'curriculum of life' that served them before serving the system or the economy; his *scientific competence* shown in his rigorous and robust intellectual preparation which eventually translated into a major resource in a resourceless educational site; and his *joy of living* exhibited in his resistance to a 'necrophilic' conception of life informed by helplessness, fatalism and resignation in relation to a profoundly unjust world.

The transformative educator, as exemplified by don Milani, is recognised by the students of Barbiana as the antidote to the school teachers that had failed them. Right from the very beginning of the *Lettera,* and throughout their collective writing effort, the student-authors attribute their predicament to teachers who lacked the social consciousness, the emotional affinity and the academic competence to be there for all children to succeed:

> You will not even remember my name. You have failed many of them.
>
> On the other hand, I have often thought of you, of your colleagues, about that institution that you call school, about the children that you "turn away".
>
> Yes, turn us away to the fields and to the factories and you forget about us. (School of Barbiana, 2009, p. 33)

Conclusion

Emancipatory nurture groups respond to a vision of education as a committed act of 'social transgression (Hooks, 1994). An education process that refuses to speak the language of individual rehabilitation, while embracing a pedagogy of mutual transformation. Such pedagogy is context-bound and is constantly reinvented and reconceptualised to serve as a catalyst for everyone within the child's ecology to become more engaged in a learning process that promotes personal and social change.

Emancipatory nurture groups foreground the concept of engaged voices that can never be fixed and absolute. Voices that evolve within a radical space of possibility and in dialogue with the world. Affirming voices within emancipatory nurture groups also implies the validation of different knowledges and ways of knowing. Cognitive justice is forged in the realisation that emancipation cannot be achieved if the members of the nurture group enter the learning community as voiceless objects of the institution's rehabilitative gaze. An emancipatory agenda informed by the valorisation and affirmation of voices, conceives of the learning communities as makers of cognition, spaces where everyone feels mutually responsible to contribute to collective emancipation and weaning from a deficit-oriented system.

Emancipatory nurture groups are learning ecologies, where parents matter. Don Milani and his students were well aware that parents could play a decisive role in the struggle for quality and equity in education. The *Lettera* directly addressed parents:

> This book is not written for teachers but for parents. It is a call to get organised. (School of Barbiana, 2009, p. 32)

Emancipatory nurture groups exist in the practicality of living in an unequal world, and thrive in a pedagogical condition that negates prescription, privileges participation, and promotes democracy; a space where knowledge is produced communally and where doubt and dissent to oppressive structures is encouraged.

Finally, emancipatory nurture groups promote mutual transformation as educators reach out not as untouchable experts but a co-creator of opportunities for students who have been often construed as unteachable.

References

Borg, C. (2022a). Parents as 'subjects'. Revisiting parent-adult educator relations in viral times, *Encyclopaideia – Journal of Phenomenology and Education, 28*(63), 56–68.

Borg, C. (2022b). When the academic 'tourist gaze' evolves into collaboration with the parent 'other': Parents as protagonists of knowledge production. In C. Borg (Ed.), *Reimagining parenthood in diverse contexts: A handbook of parent-centred approaches* (pp. 65–80). Faculty of Education, University of Malta.

Borg, C., & Mayo, P. (2006). Critical pedagogy and citizenship. In C. Borg & P. Mayo (Eds), *Learning and social difference: Challenges for public education and critical pedagogy* (pp. 129–148). Paradigm Publishers.

Borg, C., Cardona, M., & Caruana, S. (2009). *Letter to a teacher: Lorenzo Milani's contribution to critical citizenship*. Agenda.

Cooper, P. (2008). Nurturing attachment to school: Contemporary perspectives on social, behavioural and emotional difficulties. *Pastoral Care in Education, 26*(1), 13–22.

Freire, P. (1997). *Teachers as cultural workers: Letters to those who dare teach*. Westview Press.

Hooks, B. (1994). *Teaching to Transgress*. New York: Routledge.

Martinelli, A. (2007). *Don Lorenzo Milani: Dal motivo occassionale al motivo profondo*. Società Editrice Fiorentina.

Rossi, N., & Cole, T. (1970). *Letter to a teacher by the schoolboys of Barbiana*. Penguin Books.

School of Barbiana. (2009). Letter to a teacher. In C. Borg, M. Cardona, & S. Caruana (Eds), *Letter to a teacher: Lorenzo Milani's contribution to critical citizenship*. Agenda.

Simeone, D. (2009). Prologue. In C. Borg, M. Cardona, & S. Caruana (Eds), *Letter to a teacher: Lorenzo Milani's contribution to critical citizenship*. Agenda.

Toriello, F. (2008). Lettera a una professoressa quarant'anni dopo: Una lettura interculturale. In G. Abbate (Ed.), *Don Milani: Tra scuola e impegno civile*. Luciano Editore.

CORINNA BARKER AND HELEN COWIE

10 Developmental Effects on the Daughters of Absent Fathers: The Need for Nurture

Introduction

In the course of his lifelong commitment to research that would enhance the well-being of children and young people, Paul Cooper turned his attention to the impact of Nurture Groups on children who find it hard to settle in school because of emotional difficulties in their lives. He affirmed in his work the need for schools to adopt a nurturing approach, not only to the social and emotional needs of children but also to their learning. Our chapter is about a rather neglected group, the daughters of absent fathers. They tend to be overlooked and suffer in silence. Paul's positive evaluations of Nurture Groups were, we felt, very relevant to this group of children, especially as Nurture Groups have now evolved into a whole-school nurture approach. Our chapter is, we hope, a tribute to the thoughtful, sensitive, humane stance which permeates his work and remains as his legacy.

Background

Across Europe divorce rates have increased, so that more children are living without both parents in their households than in the past (Auersperg et al., 2019). Furthermore, it has been found that on average children find it more difficult to talk to their fathers about social and emotional aspects of their lives compared to their mothers (UNICEF,

2013). The combination of reduced time and communication difficulties indicates that the relationships fathers have with their children are put under a lot of pressure following physical separation.

Father absence refers to the situation where a child has lived part, or all, of their childhood in a house without their biological father, with the effects of this felt not only during childhood, but in adolescence and adulthood as well (Mancini, 2010; Zirima, 2019). Research to date in this area tends to have its focus on the father-son dyad, with literature describing how boys with absent fathers can 'become victims of their undeciphered fears, and how these fears are manifested in the deprivation syndrome Herzog has labelled "father hunger"' (Rubin, 2002, p. 698). A much smaller body of research focuses on the impact of father absence on daughters. Even fewer studies examine support mechanisms that could benefit girls at earlier stages in their lifespan in overcoming the difficulties they may face through having an absent father. Father absence often comes with a sense of abandonment on the part of the daughter (Castetter, 2020) with such long-term effects as poor academic attainment, lower self-esteem, internalised feelings of rejection, and a greater likelihood of depression and anxiety during childhood and adolescence. There is some evidence too that girls experience identity struggles as a direct impact of father abandonment, with the loss of this relationship potentially shaping future interactions with males (Perkins, 2001).

Father-Child Attachment

From the perspective of attachment theory, some researchers (e.g. Freeman et al., 2010; Suess et al., 1992; van IJzendoorn & Wolff, 1997) view the role of fathers in a child's social and emotional development as 'additive' to the role of mothers, implying that father-child attachment types are not as significant. Others argue that father and mother attachment relationships derive from different sets of early social experiences, with the father providing security through sensitive and challenging support as a play partner when the child's exploratory system is aroused (e.g.

Dumont & Paquette, 2012; Leidy et al., 2013). Activation relationship theory refers to 'the triggering of emotional arousal mechanisms stimulated by exposure to new experiences, or strangeness – an essential step in the development of social competencies' (Paquette, 2004, p. 203). From this perspective, by encouraging children to explore a stimulating outside environment, while providing discipline by setting limits for their safety, fathers establish an affectional bond that is needed in the development of children's sense of security and self-confidence.

The Fatherhood Institute (2012, p. 1) reports that not having a supportive relationship with one's biological father (resident or non-resident) is a major risk factor for youth drug and alcohol abuse, mental health challenges, educational failure, anti-social behaviour and difficult transitions into adult relationships. Stereotypes surrounding gender roles and masculinity still exist within society and family contexts, hindering the extent to which absent fathers may be actively involved in their children's lives.

According to Maine (2010), father hunger is a deep persistent desire for an emotional connection with the father, which, if it is not addressed, continues into adulthood with this longing brought into focus in the formation of new relationships. This could explain why girls and young women who have absent fathers often crave male attention, with findings suggesting that some may cling on to their romantic partner due to fear of abandonment (Peyper, 2013), while others avoid deep commitment by engaging in casual sex and short-term relationships. Recent research suggests that the lack of a father-daughter relationship leads to girls' distorted perception of males, particularly in the context of intimate relationships (Castetter, 2020; Krauss et al., 2019). Salmon et al. (2016), in their study of the impact of father absence on college students' engagement in casual sex, found that the earlier the students were no longer living with their biological father, the more they engaged in casual sex and one-night stands. At the same time, the young women exhibited more concerns than the men about casual sex as well as wondering about their partners' intentions and feelings. However, there is a lack of empirical research isolating emotional and psychological components of father hunger from father presence and father absence (Perrin et al., 2009). Children are assumed to have father hunger if they have absent fathers despite never being assessed for it and relationships are assumed to have existed without research documenting such relationships. From this, it is evident that exploration of father hunger in daughters is required for a more in-depth understanding of the impact on girls.

The Impact of Father Absence on Girls' Self Esteem

Self-esteem has been shown to predict relationship satisfaction, job success and physical health, with research suggesting that the early childhood family environment has long-term effects on self-esteem which can still be observed in adulthood (Krauss et al., 2019). Research shows that father involvement is associated with increased self-confidence and higher self-esteem through encouragement of environmental exploration and risk-taking (Hill et al., 2016). This can be linked back to theories of father-child attachment types, such as the activation relationship theory, as it supports the idea that an active and playful relationship between a father and daughter creates a bond that helps a child build self-confidence. It is evident that early father-daughter relationships play an important role in the development of high self-esteem and confidence amongst girls, which can impact many aspects of life and overall wellbeing. However, findings have shown that a consistent relationship with the mother and closeness to grandparents are statistically significant in supporting the development of resilience when faced with difficulties (Napora, 2019). Such qualities can be used to overcome challenges such as self-acceptance and confidence amongst father-absent daughters.

The present research explored the following questions: What impact does early father absence have on girls' social and emotional development? What impact does early father absence have on adolescent/early adult relationships? What can be done to support fatherless girls in overcoming the social and emotional impact of having an absent father?

Methodology

In an online survey, participants were asked to reflect on personal experiences of father absence during childhood and how this impacted them personally as adolescents/young adults. This method ensured confidentiality and anonymity since participants were not required to communicate directly with the researcher. Such a survey methodology generates both quantitative and qualitative findings, asking both open ended and closed questions. The selection criteria for the participants were as follows: all identified as women; they were over the age of 18; they had experienced a prolonged father absence as children.

Due to the nature of the study, participants were not asked their age as this was not relevant to the research. However, confirmation of respondents being 18 years or older was required before they completed the survey. The research took account of ethical guidelines (BERA, 2018) showing an ethic of respect for the person, knowledge, democratic values, the quality of educational research, and academic freedom, and was approved by the Liverpool Hope University Ethics Committee. This was done by stating the aims of the research, while ensuring the safety and privacy of participants and reducing risks through the guarantee of confidentiality and anonymity.

The questionnaire comprised fifteen questions with each section having an open text qualitative question to record further thoughts and observations. This chapter discusses the questions that considered social and emotional aspects of development. There were fifty participants, all female, who were recruited by posting the survey on social media pages which generated responses quickly. Each participant had experienced prolonged father absence during her childhood years. Reasons for the absence included death of the father, divorce from the mother, father living abroad, father serving a lengthy prison sentence, father never known (Table 10.1). The age at which father began is shown in Table 10.2.

Table 10.1. Participants' explanations for the absence of the father

Separation/divorce	56%
Death of the father	8%
Father never involved/working abroad	8%
Father in prison	4%
Prefer not to say	2%
Other	22%

Table 10.2. Reported ages of participants when father became absent

Age	Percentage of Sample
Before birth	12%
6–10 years	44%
11–15 years	14%
16 or over	4%

Thematic analysis was used to examine the findings, which is a 'method for systematically identifying, organising and offering insight into patterns of meaning across a data set' (Braun & Clarke, 2012, p. 57). The thematic analysis of the qualitative data was conducted manually. Coding was generated from thematic patterns emerging from the data. Themes were reviewed and revised with nine distinct themes emerging. The results of the thematic analysis are summarised in Table 10.3.

Table 10.3. Themes that emerged from the participants' responses

Research Question	Themes
What impact does early father absence have on girls' social and emotional development?	1. Deep feelings of sadness 2. Father hunger 3. Idealisation of the absent father 4. Perceptions of social pressure to have a father in your life
What impact does early father absence have on adolescent/early adult relationships?	5. Lack of trust in men/fear of abandonment 6. Lower self-esteem

Research Question	Themes
What can be done to support fatherless girls in overcoming the social and emotional impact of having an absent father?	7. Critical role of mother and other family members 8. Importance of positive male role models 9. Lack of support and understanding at school

Results

What Impact Does Early Father Absence Have on Girls' Social and Emotional Development?

Respondents were asked to reflect on the impact of father absence during childhood, adolescence and adulthood through questions such as 'what was it like not having a father during your childhood?' and 'as an adult, what feelings do you associate with your father?' In answer to the first research question, four main themes emerged: Deep feelings of sadness; father hunger; idealisation of the absent father; and perceptions of social pressure to have a father in your life.

Deep feelings of sadness. The research literature (as summarised by Castetter, 2020) indicates that fatherless children often report sadness when they observe other children having positive experiences with their fathers. The responses of participants in the present study confirmed this finding. They frequently described the sadness they felt in childhood when seeing their peers interacting in playful and affectionate ways with their fathers. One respondent wrote:

> 'I really wanted the connection with a father like I saw my friends have.'

Another stated:

> 'I felt sad seeing other kids my age celebrating Father's Day'.

Father hunger. Closely related to the theme of sadness and in line with the concept of 'father hunger' were reports of longings to be with the absent father. The concept of father hunger describes a deep persistent desire for an emotional connection with the father (Maine, 2010). Many of the women expressed their yearning for the father who was not in her life. But they also expressed anger and disappointment that they could not relate to him. One participant who had experienced father absence since her pre-school years wrote that she felt many conflicting emotions about her father which continued into adulthood. As an adult, she associated feelings of stress, disappointment and confusion with her father, stating that she and her father 'rarely ever speak but I still put a lot of weight in his approval, and worry about what he might think'. She added:

> 'I am apprehensive about wanting a relationship with my father.' /

Similarly, one respondent reported that:

> 'I went through desperation years trying to get a meaningful connection with him (father)'.

Idealisation of the absent father. Some reported that they had few or no memories of their father. Consequently, they 'didn't know anything else' and 'it didn't have much impact at the time'. Others, however, wrote that they had created an idealised picture of what their father might be like:

> 'I think I slightly glamourised what it would be like to have a dad in my head.'

Another wrote:

> 'I really wanted the connection – a father – like I saw my friends have or like in films.'

This confirms Witten (2017) who interpreted this phenomenon as a form of mourning for the loss of a father.

Perceptions of social pressure to have a father. Even though the incidence of families without fathers is on the increase in Western society, the women in the present study still experienced a strong sense that their family was 'different' or 'lacking' in some way, indicating the persistence of the belief that the nuclear family is the norm. This implies that the social expectations of society put pressure on girls to conform to fit social norms. One respondent wrote:

> 'It was not socially acceptable to have a broken home'.

Furthermore, the social constructions of fatherhood and paternal involvement with children have changed over time, shifting from the father as mainly breadwinner, to a more child-centred role (Mavungu, 2013). This change could exacerbate feelings of societal pressures on father absent girls (Fatherhood Institute, 2012). This shift within society may lead to girls feeling that they *ought* to have a relationship with their father. As one participant put it:

> 'I feel as though I am expected to form a bond with him.'

These findings suggest that researchers need to look beyond the father-daughter relationship (or its absence) to explore wider social constructions o fathering roles.

What Impact Does Early Father Absence Have on Adolescent/Young Adult Relationships?

In answer to the second research question, two themes emerged: Lack of trust in men/fear of abandonment and lower self-esteem.

Lack of trust in men/fear of abandonment. The qualitative data collected from the present survey confirm vulnerability regarding intimacy with men, with thirty-six participants reporting that father absence affected romantic relationships. Several respondents also stated their fear of abandonment and insecurities in romantic relationships, indicating support for the concept of *father hunger*, despite the negative associations they held of him.

> 'I found it difficult to talk to men.'
>
> 'I find it hard to trust men, so it makes relationships hard.'
>
> 'I fear abandonment.'

'I do not want to rely on anyone too much.'

'I have an anxious attachment in most of my relationships.'

While none of the participants gave detailed accounts of their romantic/sexual relationships, a consistent theme was anxiety that their partners would abandon them and persistent difficulties in maintaining intimate relationships with men.

Lower self-esteem. Thirty two reported that their self-esteem had been affected. Typical responses were:

'It's something that influenced my self-esteem in a negative way.'

'My self-worth is very low.'

'I have low self-esteem; I think this started with the feelings of unworthiness as a child.'

These findings confirmed activation relationship theory (Dumont & Paquette, 2012), which proposes that the encouragement of exploration and risk-taking play with fathers in early life strengthens the paternal affectional bond and so leads to higher self-esteem amongst offspring (Hill et al., 2016). From this perspective, the role of the father is vital. The way a father interacts with his daughter shapes her self-image and mental health (Del Russo, 2009), explaining why fatherless daughters experience low self-esteem, as a lack of encouragement from a father may lead to self-doubt and the feelings of unworthiness.

What Can Be Done to Support Fatherless Girls in Overcoming the Emotional and Social Impact of Having an Absent Father?

In answer to the third research question, three themes emerged: Critical role of mother and other family members; importance of positive male role models; and lack of support and understanding at school.

Critical role of mothers and other family members. Responses indicated the value of positive role modelling and coping mechanisms on the part of mothers (see Napora, 2019; Zulu, 2014) when faced with difficulties around father absence. In the present study, twenty-nine participants stated that their mother helped them cope with having an absent father. One respondent wrote:

> 'I don't think having a strong male presence is the be all and end all, but having a strong parental figure is very important'.

Another wrote:

> 'It is more important that the child is brought up by one good parent than two who cannot get on together'.

Similarly, one participant wrote:

> 'She (mother) taught me everything I need to know and really set a good example as a single mum ... she really is my idol'.

Importance of positive male role models. The findings also highlight the importance of having positive male role models, often from the family (e.g. a grandfather or uncle) or from the community (e.g. a friendly shop owner or a family friend).

One participant reported:

> 'There were family members who helped me with my daily tasks'.

These role models were not necessarily male:

> 'Having adult role models of both genders is important'.

The contradictions in responses give weight to the argument of father absence being a complex issue, as it highlights individual differences and opinions on the role of other family and community members. Significantly, in the present study, none of the women mentioned male teachers as positive role models.

The lack of support and understanding at school. Only five participants reported receiving support from school. With much of the child development literature looking at mother-child relationships, teachers may not be aware of the long-term impact on girls' social and emotional wellbeing, resulting in limited support within educational settings (Leidy et al., 2013;

Morell-Velasco et al., 2020). Additionally, there are persistent issues of stigma surrounding father absence, which may lead to teachers ignoring the impact father absence can have on their students. Krohn and Bogan (2001) proposed that fatherless girls fall into one of two categories, either overachieving or underachieving, highlighting the importance of teacher support to ensure girls are fulfilling their potential on all fronts, academic, social and emotional, despite the difficulties they may face as a result of father absence. Willemse (2018, p. 252) argues that the 'collaboration between educational institutions, teachers and families can influence pupils' and students' academic achievements, social development and sense of wellbeing in all levels of education'. This raises concern around the findings from the survey, due to such a small number of respondents saying they received support in school, despite the literature highlighting the important role school plays in supporting children and families in this situation.

The majority of participants said receiving support during their own childhood would have benefitted them though acknowledging that it would not be helpful to have attention drawn to their situation. A typical response was:

> 'It would also be important that the girls were not made to feel different (yet again) from families with both parents'.

This raises the risk that support groups, if carried out in an insensitive way, might stigmatise fatherless girls further, which could lead to additional self-esteem and confidence issues. For example, Wood and Brownhill (2018) caution that when male teachers take on the role of 'replacement fathers', there is the risk of engaging in parental blame which in turn may be emotionally damaging to the child.

Another participant addresses this concern by stating the value of sensitive understanding by teachers:

> 'Normalising talking about feelings and not making children feel guilty/told off for getting upset and angry'.

Discussion

The nuclear family model is still considered as the norm within society, despite the seemingly progressive reform and acceptance of a greater variety of family forms and the fact that fatherless families are increasingly common in Western society (Brown, 2019). This raises the question of whether a shift in trends and norms within society regarding the structure of family is needed to reduce the social and emotional impacts of father absence, rather than support that focuses specifically on the individual child, which may lead to girls feeling further stigmatised. 'Family ideals shape the available cultural repertoire through which actual men and women talk about, and think about, their own family lives' (Edgell & Docka, 2007, p. 26), explaining why girls may feel pressures from society to form a relationship with their father and to conform to the ideal of the nuclear family.

The results of the present study point to two broad ways in which schools can alleviate some of the emotional difficulties experienced by girls whose fathers are absent, for whatever reason. On the one hand, schools have the opportunity to challenge stereotypical views on the nature of the family, while on the other hand, they can help individual girls to deal with social and emotional issues that have arisen as a result of father absence. Educators can address negative attitudes towards parents who do not conform to the traditional family model without focusing specifically on a particular student in their class and certainly, whether explicitly or implicitly, should not blame single mothers or absent fathers for their children's social and emotional difficulties. Instead, we argue, it is more constructive to move away from a 'deficit' model of parenting to one that takes account of societal constraints, such as poverty or social isolation, that make parenting difficult. A more productive model involves a cooperative exchange between parents and teachers. Rather than focusing only on girls who do not have fathers, society as a whole must change (Mavungu, 2013; Wood & Brownhill, 2018). The normalisation of father absence in society may lead to girls not feeling 'worthless', 'unloved' and having a 'fear of abandonment', which could lead to the long-term negative impacts on self-esteem, relationships and achievement being reduced, due to father absence not holding such a negative connotation within society. At the same time, more needs to be done through the SEL curriculum in addressing the needs of girls with absent fathers in ways that do not further stigmatise them. In tandem, educators can develop a supportive climate throughout the school in which relationships of trust and nurturance are valued and enhanced in all aspects of school life.

One innovative approach, developed by Marjorie Boxall (Boxall & Lucas, 2010) and grounded in attachment theory, comes from the development of Nurture Groups (NGs) which focus on the need for children to form secure and happy relationships with others during their formative years, particularly for those children who have missed out in some way, for example, through the absence of a father, on the experiences that promote positive, trusting relationships with peers and adults, (in the present case, particularly males). NG teachers are trained to understand the emotional issues that affect these children and to meet their needs through the creation of a safe, secure and supportive environment. NG provision helps children and adolescents to address both internalising and externalising behavioural difficulties. Most importantly, NG provision is distinctive in the length of time involved in helping children to form strong trusting relationships with adults who show them affection, give them attention and reassure them of their self-worth and personal value. In essence, the targeted intervention of the small supportive NG creates a safe space that bridges the gap between home and school by providing opportunities to recreate the missed early experiences (such as the experience of father presence) through trusting, nurturing relationships with specially trained teachers. This involves identifying and understanding individual students' social, emotional and mental health needs and helping them to gain insights into their relationships with others.

However, more recently, many schools are also adopting a whole school nurturing approach, using Boxall's six nurture principles for learning as a method for helping all children and young people to develop social skills, confidence and self-esteem (Nurture International, 2023):

- Learning and achievement is enhanced through meeting social, emotional, and cognitive needs.
- How we communicate impacts on mental health, learning and achievement.
- Nurture cultures promote reflective practices.
- Self-esteem and a sense of identity are key to positive mental health and wellbeing.
- Feeling emotionally safe is essential for mental health, learning and achievement.
- Celebration of diversity enriches the community and enhances learning.

Evaluations of NGs (Cooper & Whitebread, 2007; Middleton, 2022; Scott Loinaz, 2015) indicate significant gains in children's self-esteem, emotional maturity, resilience, emotional literacy skills, and in their capacity to engage with others and to form closer attachments with them. Such experiences would provide the kind of understanding and emotional support that the daughters of absent fathers so desperately needed during their childhood years, as shown in the present study.

Conclusion

This study has generated important findings in an under-researched area – the impact of early father absence – confirming some of the findings in the field while questioning others. A particular contribution to the issue that is raised is the importance of providing an alternative stance through empathic nurturing of fatherless girls, with NGs or a whole-school nurturing approach in schools being key examples of how such support might be done in a sensitive, child-centred way.

The concept of fatherhood is in a process of being redefined as society changes and the roles of men and women evolve. The findings of the present study confirm the view that fathers play a significant role in their daughters' social and emotional development and that their absence is likely to have a strong impact on girls' future relationships with men through adolescence into adulthood. In light of the increasing numbers of fatherless families, it is essential for us to know more about the outcomes for both fatherless girls and for the men who miss out on the experience of raising their daughters.

Limitations of the Study

Despite there being many advantages of an online survey, there are also disadvantages. Although carrying out a survey online means participants from all locations can respond, there is a risk that people who do not have access to the internet or are under confident in using online pages will not take part. This has been referred to as the 'digital divide' between people who have internet access and people who do not (Curtis et al., 2014; Morison et al., 2015). The issue of misremembering feelings and emotion is something that the researcher must be cognisant of as past feelings may be reconstructed by beliefs about how we should feel, with there often being biases towards the most intense emotion felt at the time (Urban et al., 2019). Furthermore, research has suggested our 'first memories' are reconstructions based on family stories and photographs (Milton, 2018), implying that memories can be modified when retelling experiences, leading to inaccuracies in what a person remembers.

References

Auersperg, F., Vlasak, T., Ponocny, I., & Barth, A. (2019). Long term effects of parental divorce on mental health – A meta-analysis. *Journal of Psychiatric Research, 119,* 107–115.
Boxall, M., & Lucas, S. (Eds) (2010). *Nurture groups in schools* (2nd edn). Sage.
Braun, V., & Clarke, V. (2012). Thematic analysis. *Qualitative Research in Clinical and Health Psychology, 24*(95), 57–71.
British Educational Research Association (BERA). (2018). *Ethical guidelines for educational research* (4th edn). <https://www.bera.ac.uk/researchers-resources/publications/ethical-guidelines-for-educational-research-2018>

Brown, A. (2019). *What is the family of law? The influence of the nuclear family.* Bloomsbury Publishing.

Castetter, C. (2020). The developmental effects on the daughter of an absent father throughout her lifespan. *Merrimack Scholar Works, 50,* 1–20. <https://scholarworks.merrimack.edu/honors_capstones/50>

Cooper, P., & Whitebread, D. (2007). The effectiveness of nurture groups on student progress: Evidence from a national research study. *Emotional and Behavioural Difficulties, 12*(3), 171–190.

Curtis, W., Murphy, W., Shields, S., & Murphy, M. (2014). *Research and education.* Routledge.

Del Russo, J. (2009). *Emotionally absent fathers and their adult daughters' relationship with men.* Chestnut Hill College: Pro Quest Dissertations Publishing.

Dumont, C., & Paquette, D. (2012). What about the child's tie to the father? A new insight into fathering, father-child attachment, children's socio-emotional development and the activation theory. *Early Childhood Development and Care, 183*(3), 430–446.

Edgell, P., & Docka, D. (2007). Beyond the nuclear family? Familism and gender ideology in diverse religious communities. *Sociological Forum, 22*(1), 25–50.

Fatherhood Institute. (2012). *Addressing fatherlessness: How government can strengthen the active presence of fathers in their children's lives.* <http://www.fatherhoodinstitute.org/2012/addressing-fatherlessness-a-fatherhood-institute-policy-briefing/>

Freeman, H., Newland, L., & Coyl, D. (2010). New directions in father attachment. *Early Childhood Development and Care, 180*(1), 1–8.

Hill, S. E., Leyva, R. P. P., & DelPriore, D. (2016). Absent fathers and sexual strategies. *The Psychologist, 29*(6), 436–439.

Krauss, S., Orth, U., & Robins, R. (2019). Family environment and self-esteem development: A longitudinal study from age 10 to 16. *Journal of Personality and Social Psychology, 119*(2), 457–478.

Krohn, F., & Bogan, Z. (2001). The effect absent fathers have on female development and college attendance. *College Student Journal, 35*(4), 598–608.

Leidy, M., Schofield, T., & Parke, R. (2013). Fathers' contributions to children's social development. In N. Cabrera & C. Tamis-LeMonda (Eds), *Handbook of father involvement* (2nd edn) (pp. 151–167). Routledge.

Maine, M. (2010). *Father hunger: Fathers, daughters, and the pursuit of thinness* (2nd edn) Gurze Books.

Mancini, L. (2010). Father absence and its effects on daughters. *Ohio Family Rights, 1*(37), 1–37.

Mavungu, E. (2013). Provider expectations and father involvement: Learning from experiences of poor 'absent fathers' in Gauteng, South Africa. *African Sociological Review, 17*(1), 65–78.

Middleton, A. (2022). The nurtureuk violence reduction unit programme: Exploring a model for reducing school exclusions and instances of youth violence through nurture practice. *International Journal of Nurture in Education, 8,* 67–87.

Milton, A. (2018). The mis(remembrance) of things past: Mechanisms of memory storage, updating and why we misremember. *The Biochemist, 40*(5), 4–8.

Morell-Velasco, C., Fernandez-Alcantara, M., Hueso-Montoro, C., & Montoya-Juarez, R. (2020). Teachers' perceptions of grief in primary and secondary school students in Spain: Children's responses and elements which facilitate or hinder the grieving process. *Journal of Pediatric Nursing, 51*(1), 100–107.

Morison, T., Gibson, A., Wigginton, B., & Crabb, S. (2015). Online research methods in psychology: Methodological opportunities for critical qualitative research. *Qualitative Research in Psychology, 12*(3), 223–232.

Napora, E. (2019). Relationship with the mother and closeness to grandparents in relation to resilience in adolescents in families of single mothers. Significance of the absence of the father. *Archives of Psychiatry and Psychotherapy, 21*(4), 62–71.

Nurture International. (2023). *The six nurture principles for learning.* <https://www.nurtureinternational.co.uk>

Paquette, D. (2004). Theorizing the father-child relationship: Mechanism and developmental outcomes. *Human Development, 47*(4), 193–219.

Perkins, R. (2001). The father daughter relationship: Familial interactions that impact a daughter's style of life. *College Student Journal, 35*(4), 616–627.

Perrin, P., Baker, J., Romelus, A., Jones, K., & Heesacker, M. (2009). Development, validation, and confirmatory factor analysis of the Father Hunger Scale. *Psychology of Men and Masculinity, 10*(4), 314–327.

Peyper, E. (2013). Experiences of young adult women with emotionally absent fathers. *Journal of Psychology in Africa, 25*(2), 127–133.

Rubin, L. S. (2002). Book review: Father hunger: Explorations with adults and children. *Journal of American Psychoanalytic Association, 50*(2), 698–701.

Salmon, C., Townsend, J. M., & Hehman, J. (2016). Casual sex and college students: Sex differences and the impact of father absence. *Evolutionary Psychological Science, 2,* 254–226.

Scott Loinaz, E. (2015). Comparing nurture group provision with one-to-one counselling: What characteristics and evidence-based components produce positive change? *International Journal of Nurture in Education, 1*(1), 25–32.

Suess, G. J., Grossman, K. E., & Sroufe, L. (1992). Effects on infant attachment to mother and father on quality of adaptation in preschool: From dyadic to individual organisation of self. *International Journal of Behavioural Development, 15*(1), 43–65.

UNICEF Office of Research. (2013). Child wellbeing in rich countries: A comparative overview. *Innocenti Report Card 11*. UNICEF Office of Research.

Urban, E., Cochran, K., Acevedo, A., Cross, M., Pressman, S., & Loftus, E. (2019). Misremembering pain: A memory blindness approach to adding a better end. *Memory & Cognition, 47*(5), 954–967.

van IJzendoorn, M. H., & Wolff, M. S. (1997). In search of the absent father – meta-analyses of infant-father attachment: A rejoinder to our discussants. *Child Development, 68*(4), 604–609.

Willemse, T., Thompson, I., Vanderlinde, R., & Mutton, R. (2018). Family school partnerships: A challenge or teacher education. *Journal of Education for Teaching, 44*(3), 252–257.

Witten, M. (2017). A child mourns the family he cannot come from. *Psychoanalytic Inquiry, 37*(8), 549–554.

Wood, P., & Brownhill, S. (2018). 'Absent fathers', and children's social and emotional learning: An exploration of the perceptions of 'positive male role models' in the primary school sector. *Gender and Education, 30*(2), 172–186.

Zirima, H. (2019). *Subjective wellbeing among women with father absence experience in Masvingo: Depression, anxiety and relationship strategy*, Unpublished PhD thesis, Julius Nyerere School of Social Sciences, Great Zimbabwe University.

Zulu, N. (2014). *'I am making it without you, dad!': Fatherless female students*. Master's Thesis. University of KwaZulu-Natal.

PART IV

Engaging Students with Social, Emotional and Behavioural Difficulties

KATE WINCHESTER AND CHRIS FORLIN

11 Overcoming Disengagement of Students through an Arts-Based Programme

Introduction

Prior extensive research by Paul Cooper while in Hong Kong, with data from 914 teachers and 573 parents of children with social-emotional/behavioural problems, found a range of specific behavioural issues (Forlin & Cooper, 2013). The most frequently reasons cited by both teachers and parents were the students' lack of motivation, difficulty in facing failure, and the student getting overexcited. Such high levels of student problems in educational engagement, motivation, cooperation, and oppositionality, were considered highly problematic not only for the students, but were also considered as emotional triggers for their teachers and parents. Based on this evidence, an alternative approach to improving student motivation and positive engagement was designed using an arts-based pedagogy that provided an authentic platform for disadvantaged students to engage in learning in a more positive and rewarding way. This chapter presents an action research project with students from three disadvantaged communities in Australia, investigating the relationship between student engagement, creativity, social-emotional learning, and arts-based pedagogical approaches.[1]

---

1 This chapter draws partly from the first author's unpublished PhD thesis: Winchester, K. (2015). *'No kid is an island': The Gallery as a classroom space for creativity, student engagement and the bigger pictures.* Unpublished thesis submitted at Western Sydney University, Australia.

Background

Classrooms within schools from low socio-economic (SES) areas, are often characterised by ranging levels of complex factors such as disruptive student resistance, low-learner self-concept, fractured student or community relationships with mainstream society, reductive teaching practices, negative media attention for the school community, high student mobility, and specific student cultural needs (Sawyer & Munns, 2019). The complexities at work in these schools contribute toward maintaining restrictive pedagogies and are driven by high-pressure educational systems (Riddle et al., 2021; Sawyer & Munns, 2019). Within this context, it raises the question of how potentially disadvantaged students from low SES areas can engage fully in education and meet equitable outcomes.

The backgrounds of students from low SES schools are frequently viewed in deficit ways with the consequence that expectations are lowered, and the curriculum is constricted (Hernandez et al., 2021). Such consequences can elucidate why many students from low SES backgrounds disengage from schooling.

International schooling policies indicate that there is a severe gap in educational outcomes for disadvantaged communities (Sawyer & Munns, 2019; Program for International Student Assessment (PISA)). This trend is intensified through western educational policy, that has focused on test-based accountability, market-oriented reform ideas such as competition between schools, a prescribed curriculum, the focus on literacy and numeracy, and standardised teaching practices (Baldacchino, 2019). According to Lingard (2013) '… any focus on disadvantaged students from poor communities and their school is framed by this test-driven accountability and likely to limit the intellectual demands made on students, exacerbating inequality in and through schooling' (p. xi). The dominating pedagogy in such classrooms can invariably be defined in terms of teacher control, restricted curriculum, and practices that foster comparison and competition, driven from performative measures (Sawyer & Munns, 2019). In this paper it is argued that students in all classrooms, particularly those in disadvantaged contexts, deserve engaging and meaningful learning experiences.

Overcoming Disengagement of Students

Arts-based learning, or the intentional use of artistic skills and processes as tools to enhance learning outcomes in non-artistic disciplines, was the pedagogical vehicle that was adopted as part of the research design. By adopting arts-based learning as the foundation of the design of the learning programs, the research investigates whether this can provide an authentic platform for disadvantaged students to engage in learning about the world around them, through examining big ideas of human significance and impact. In focusing on the critical gap in educational outcomes for students living in low SES, it aims to reflect ethical and moral reasons to support disadvantaged communities educationally through more appropriate pedagogy for engagement.

Student Engagement

The relationship between teachers and students has been a key determinant in supporting the engagement of learners (Allen et al., 2018; Munns, 2021). Developing a positive relationship is especially critical when endeavouring to engage students who demonstrate behavioural challenges, are uninspired, or disenfranchised by learning, and lack empathy for others. According to Forlin and Cooper (2013):

> Teachers who show warmth, empathy, and respect for students and create a nurturing environment are, nonetheless, likely to prevent the development of disruptive behaviour and encourage positive self-regard and pro-social engagement among students. (p. 58)

Extensive research by Paul Cooper while in Hong Kong, with data from 914 teachers and 573 parents of children with social-emotional/behavioural problems, found a range of responses (Forlin & Cooper, 2013). The most frequently cited behavioural issues for both teachers and parents were the students' lack of motivation, difficulty in facing failure, and the child getting overexcited. Such substantial levels of student problems in relation to educational engagement, motivation, cooperativeness, and oppositionality, were considered highly problematic not only for the students, but were also emotional triggers for their teachers and parents.

Social-emotional Learning

Dewey suggests that it is highly important for students to value and see connections in their learning for '... there is no defect in traditional education greater than its failure to secure the active cooperation of the pupil in construction of the purposes involved in his studying' (1938, p. 67). Producing ideas, risk-taking, and attempting challenging tasks are often avoided by students from low SES areas (Munns, 2021), and that a more culturally responsive pedagogy would ensure safe and supportive environments as well as engaging message systems (Garrett & MacGill, 2021) These practices would encourage students to '... feel confident to take risks' and would '... promote imaginative and creative thinking and the exploration of multiple possibilities' (Arthur & Hertzberg, 2013, p. 152).

The outcome of integrating big ideas within curriculum has been seen as important to achieving social justice aims and equity when students are given work of intellectual quality and 'real world' knowledge. This approach challenges educators to focus on schooling as an intensely social and moral process, to develop a deep emotional connection between the learner and what was being learned.

Arts-Based Pedagogy

By its very nature, arts pedagogy is vastly social and can be characterised as a communal practice, playful, affective, emotive, and aesthetic, as well as intellectual (Almqvist & Vist, 2019). Two important human capacities that can be achieved through the arts pedagogical approach are empathy and imagination (Egan, 2019). Artistic pedagogy has been valued as a procedure to generate critical and evaluative thinking, and emotive and affective representation. Imaginative pedagogy can also incite critical thinking about issues of human impact (Winchester, 2021). Imagination and empathy are recognised as core human capacities and were thus promoted though arts learning as central pedagogical concerns.

Creativity

Creative pedagogy has the potential to improve the learning of students through a diverse range of skills from encouraging imaginative thinking (Egan, 2007, 2019), play and possibility thinking (Craft, 2012; Burnard & Loughrey, 2021) collaboration (Halverson & Sawyer, 2022), to critical and creative thinking (Siburia et al., 2019). This creative classroom rhetoric aligns strongly with classrooms serving low SES communities when pedagogy is employed that allows students to use imaginative thinking, inquiry, artistic and creative expression (Halverson & Sawyer, 2022; Winchester, 2021; Riddle et al., 2021; Sawyer & Munns, 2019). The links between creativity and learning can be situated in terms of a positive aspiration to improve the experience of education for disadvantaged students.

Arts-Based Research

The term 'arts-based research' is attributed to Eisner (Barone & Eisner, 2012), who sought to connect projects of social inquiry with the role of artistry. Arts-based research confronts and documents complex and subtle human interactions in order to provide rich understandings of an aspect of an experience (Barone & Eisner, 2012, p. 3). This form of research is embedded in aesthetic forms to express meanings that cannot otherwise be communicated through discursive means. Its intention is not to offer complete 'truth' but to raise further questions and ignite purposeful debate (Barone & Eisner, 2012, p. 166).

Fair Go Program (FGP)

This research is greatly informed by and takes up the social justice and equity intentions of the student engagement framework of the Fair Go Program (FGP) (Munns & Sawyer, 2013). The FGP was the outcome of an initial action research project into student engagement in low SES areas in Australia. The FGP framework, which was empirically and theoretically developed, illustrates the position that student engagement is dependent on the pedagogical relationship between teachers and students (Munns & Sawyer, 2013; Sawyer et al., 2018). It places emphasis on learning, rather than focusing on the control of student behaviour, to explore pedagogies that inspire 'in task' (substantive engagement – that is, strong psychological investment), not 'on task' (procedural engagement – that is merely complying with teacher directions) (Munns et al., 2013). This important distinction considers a broad characteristic of low SES classrooms as their pedagogical environments are often marked by the concentration on behaviour management and 'back to basics' instruction (Cole et al., 2013, p. 123) Rather than emphasising procedural engagement, the FGP focuses on substantive engagement.

Conceptual Framework

The Student Engagement Framework from The Fair Go Program (2013) was adopted to guide the pedagogy and analysis of the learning programs within this study. 'Fair go' is a familiar term in the Australian vernacular that captures an appeal to give someone 'a chance'. This research was designed to provide new ways of giving disengaged students equal 'chances' to participate in quality education and was largely influenced by the FGP student engagement framework (Figure 11.1).

This circular diagram illustrates how authentic student engagement relies on the interdependence of each element. The inner circle of the Framework represents the connection between high cognitive (thinking hard), high affective (feeling good), and high operative (becoming better learners) dimensions of experience.

Overcoming Disengagement of Students

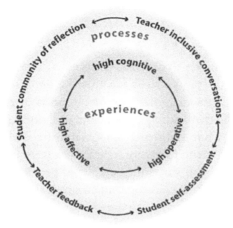

Figure 11.1. Student engagement framework (Munns, 2021, p. 3)

Classroom experiences that work towards student engagement in this model are thus those that are intellectually challenging (high cognitive), enjoyable and seen as valuable by the students (affective), and that assist them in being better learners (operative). The outer circle in the Framework includes student self-assessment, teacher inclusive conversations, teacher feedback and a student community of reflection as important processes that, when operating together, support students to feel that they are valued members of a learning community. The FGP names this as the 'insider classroom' (Munns, 2021). The notion of the insider classroom was a vital feature of this research in that the pedagogical design is based on the notion that all students should have a 'vital role to play' and enact strong involvement within their classrooms and the work that they do (Munns & Sawyer, 2013). The FGP observed that 'in-task' engagement can be perceived when students extend learning beyond teacher, task, and time.

Methodology

A key research aim was to examine the quality of pedagogical practices in the Gallery in a commitment towards the premise that all students, including those from marginalised backgrounds, need to be provided with intellectually demanding and meaningful work, not only as an engagement strategy but as a matter of social justice (Munns et al., 2013). Turning away from deficit views of socially disadvantaged classrooms, the design of the lessons in this study sought to provide pedagogy of high expectations, intellectual challenge, and a supportive classroom environment (Winchester, 2021).

Central to the methodological approach for this study was action research. Action research is the combination of action, reflection, theory, and practice (Reason & Bradbury, 2008). It further acknowledges the importance of embedding research within a socio-cultural context (Brydon-Miller et al., 2003). The partly ethnographic approach of this study involved the researcher being immersed within the research site to observe and interact with the participants through lessons, discussion, and reflection (Delamont, 2002).

Arts based research (Barone & Eisner, 2012) provided the means to understand the complex and subtle human interactions, artistic representation, and emotional expressions that were the focus of the study. The analysis of the data set out to explore perceptions of meaning and to deepen purposeful debate within this discourse. The programs were planned with the research intention of engaging students in creative and artistic learning that focused on big ideas of human significance.

Data Collection

Within each of these contexts, the focus for data collection was on the pedagogy used within the arts programs and the artistic, affective, and cognitive responses of the students. It was important to carefully collect data on the students' creative and/or artistic expressions, their levels of engagement, or being 'in-task', and their relationship to learning as a human endeavour. Video recordings, photographs, voice recordings of student and teacher interviews were collected for each Gallery lesson and the final Exhibition. Data were organised and coded according to the different levels of student engagement identified from the conceptual framework.

This research used the *Student Engagement Framework* from The Fair Go Program (Munns & Sawyer, 2013) as a conceptual model from which to analyse data. The data were generated by the participants, that is the students, their classroom teacher and the researcher. In line with arts-based research and action research, the procedures used included written records of the events in each Gallery in a research journal, interviews, case-studies, focus groups, photographs and video recordings. Data collection for the case studies included direct observation and participant observation with subsequent field notes, photographic data and focus groups. These findings were notated in code and note form. Codes were generated from the four themes of the research, namely arts pedagogy, creativity, student engagement and big ideas of human significance. Within each category, several codes were generated from points of interest that related to each theme.

Research Sites

The sites for the action research were three schools in an outer-suburban Australian city. The schools were selected based on their status as a 'Priority School'. The Priority Schools program was a government initiative to provide additional funding and services to schools that were identified as serving communities with the highest concentrations of low SES status families.

This region is characterised as having a very diverse population. In 2011, the region supported 2.02 million people, with one third of this population having migrated to Australia (NSW Government, Premier & Cabinet, 2013). The schools are all serving low SES communities, and are all influenced by factors, such as high unemployment, high percentages of families living in public housing, high student mobility, low student attendance, and frequent negative media attention (Fair Go Team, 2006). Some students had English as a Second Language (ESL) needs, others were from indigenous backgrounds, and more than half had special needs in achieving literacy and numeracy outcomes (Munns et al., 2013). In all three contexts, student engagement was prioritised as an area of focus.

One classroom from each of the three schools was selected and the researcher worked alongside the class teacher to deliver a set of lessons. Three separate arts programs were taught in each of these three classrooms to explore the levels of student engagement when there is a focus on arts-based learning in tandem with a focus on real-world issues of human concern. These programs were implemented for three hours per week across twenty weeks. The teachers who were responsible for these classes were also important to the action research approach in that their reflections on the application of the conceptual framework in practice were valued. Full ethics approval to research in three different primary classrooms was obtained through Western Sydney University and the Department of Education.

Lesson Procedure

The focus on arts-based pedagogies led to the conception of 'The Gallery' as a guiding metaphorical principle for the lessons. This was designed as a model to guide the process of the implementation of the programs to stimulate students to examine big ideas in their learning. The arts-based program included artistic learning activities such as tableau (a static and silent scene in which to replicate a moment in a story); theatre games (improvisation activities to stimulate creativity, concentration, self-expression and cooperation); dramatic dance (movement that expresses emotion, narrative action or character development) and visible thinking strategies (a set of questions that can be used in analysis of visual art to scaffold and extend student thinking) (Ritchhart et al., 2011). *The Gallery* came to be the name that was applied to the learning sessions conducted with the students to illustrate ways that a classroom can be a space for artistic expression.

Each class had between twenty-five and thirty-two students and worked as a whole group to develop and create an 'Exhibition'. Linking a classroom exhibition to that which might be seen in an everyday gallery, this type of artistic culmination was seen as an authentic opportunity for students to share with their community the deep and purposeful learning that had been occurring throughout their Gallery experiences. It was thus not seen as a disconnected, one-off artistic showcase, but rather, a purposeful exhibition of the learning undertaken.

For example, one of the Galleries conducted was with a Stage 2 (Years three and four) classroom in a school with a large majority of students from migrant backgrounds. The group were studying the topic of British colonisation of Australia, and the Gallery was designed to examine the historical impact of this event by teaching the students about the Stolen Generation (a period of Australian history from the mid-1800s to the 1970s where Aboriginal children were removed from their families through Government policies). The students were led through a series of arts-based activities which led them to read and express their emotional reactions to excerpts of real-life survivors of the Stolen Generation through artistic expression.

Results

High Cognitive Engagement

The artistic and creative pedagogy was used to facilitate a high cognitive learning environment in the promotion of critical thinking, higher order questioning, and problem solving. Early in the Gallery, it appeared that the students began to express positive emotions and affective responses to the learning. In subsequent Gallery lessons, the students' understandings of the big ideas in the area of study were illustrated in their abilities to role play moments of human significance from the texts that were used. The students were also able to express their empathic understanding by drawing on their own experience and linking them to the topic. In one of the final student focus groups, a telling conversation occurred regarding the close link between high affective and high cognitive achievement:

> *Teacher: What are the benefits of being a student in these lessons? What are the good parts?*
>
> Child: Sharing our ideas. And that we can skip class and not do work.
>
> *Teacher: Did you think that you weren't doing work?*
>
> Nope, I felt like it was all fun.
>
> *Teacher: But were you not using your brain?*
>
> Children responses: You were using your brain because you were thinking of ideas and sharing them and that's how you came up with it.
>
> Well people think maybe it (the Exhibition) was just a play but then they see it and it looks, people think it's easy but when you look at it it's easy but then when you're really behind the screen and try and do it, it looks really, really, hard.
>
> Yeah, because it's just fun and it's hard because you need to concentrate and then you're just having fun, not doing work but you're still doing work.
>
> It's good that we are getting out of work but we're still doing work because we're using our brain for thinking of ideas and sharing it and if we're doing that we can concentrate and if we concentrate it will go perfect and everything will go smooth.
>
> I was just trying to say that we were still working but working with fun.
>
> It was fun and hard. That's the whole idea.

These comments from the students reinforce the view that the students did not perceive the Gallery work as trivial but that it was purposeful, that it challenged them and that they felt a strong sense of ownership and achievement over their learning. Their reflections also indicated that they were beginning to define engagement on their own terms. There appeared, to be a pedagogical shift in the students from intellectually low-level and competitive expectations, towards effective group work, meaningful expression of knowledge, and a strong sense of ownership of learning. The enhanced High Cognitive engagement was evident in the ways in which the students were embracing more opportunities for tasks that involved problem solving and critical thinking through dramatic expression, role-play, creative writing, and artful thinking.

High Affective Engagement

The sessions involved many arts-based teaching and learning strategies that appeared to become an affective 'hook' that enabled students to feel enjoyment in their experience of the Gallery. Over time, the data suggested that this developed into a deeper, more authentic level of enjoyment for students encouraging them to feel more empowered and to gain a greater sense of ownership over their learning.

With further involvement and familiarity with the Gallery pedagogy, the evidence showed that the students began to express affective responses to the learning tasks. The students reflected on the quality of their work and expressed pride in their artistic achievements. In each subsequent Gallery, the students conveyed enthusiasm in their behaviour towards the artistic and creative learning tasks and that their active involvement in each task was reward enough. In one of the final teacher interviews, a class teacher reinforced the link between the time for reflection that was allowed in the Gallery; and indicated that the students began to see the lessons themselves and the Exhibition as an intrinsic reward. The affective hook of the lessons appeared to allow students over time to focus on their achievements and growth.

There was thus a consistency across each context that students were beginning to talk about themselves and each other as capable, valued, and interdependent members of a shared learning experience. Statements from the students at each site demonstrated their recognition of growing teamworking capabilities and that they felt more intrinsic worth from learning and achieving at new tasks. They also had 'power with' the teachers. Their combined voice showed, most significantly, engaging messages of high achievement, aspiration, connection to the task as relevant to them and shared control over the Gallery experience as being played out.

High Operative Engagement

On the high operative level, a growing sense of ownership and connection to learning become apparent for some students who were otherwise experiencing difficulty with their relationship to the classroom. There were times when teacher 'control' was not required as students were seemingly so engaged and focused on the learning task. The focus on learning and student ownership of the tasks appeared to support ongoing positive engaging messages across the Gallery experience.

Most notably, the students, whilst initially quite different in their academic and social behaviours and achievements, seemed to become more engaged learners in the Gallery. One Student, who had difficulty with risk taking and who preferred to work alone, was, from early in the Gallery, showing signs of leadership during group work and, initially, experimented artistically more than other students. The Gallery sessions allowed him to 'shine' in a new way. He stood out among his classmates in the creativity he showed and became a student whom others looked to for guidance. Another student, who was uninterested in the Gallery in the first session, became more and more involved as the sessions continued. The creative routines and artistic practices seemed to give him the physical space and release he needed to stay focused and to achieve success. His contribution to class discussions and his growing desire to be involved and to control his behaviour in order to achieve the tasks was reflective of these students' engagement. Such instances indicated the high operative engagement displayed by the students, in that they were positioning themselves as active learners in the Gallery space and were feeling increasingly comfortable and willing to embrace the pedagogy of this study, towards becoming better learners.

The Interplay between High-cognitive, -affective and -operative Levels of Student Engagement

According to The Fair Go Program (FGP) (Munns, 2021), student engagement can be defined by the equal interplay between the cognitive (thinking), affective (feeling) and operative (doing) levels; that is, students are successfully involved in tasks of intellectual quality and have passionate, positive feelings about learning. It was important therefore to examine the links between the high cognitive, affective and operative levels of the arts-based program. The data in this study suggested that the Gallery process supported the students to develop, over time, more positive relationships with learning, as well as a deeper intellectual connection to the topics of study. During initial Gallery lessons, some students displayed opposition to the pedagogy by refusing to participate and expressing resistance to arts-based tasks that they had had limited experience in. This was however, overwhelmingly replaced by positive and productive responses to the remainder of the Gallery program. An important finding from this study was that students were 'in-task' (positively involved in their learning) as opposed to being 'on-task' (just complying with teacher instructions) (Munns, 2021). The data indicated that the students were eager to take risks, were actively involved in cognitively stimulating and challenging tasks; and were communicating their positive feelings about learning.

Discussion

The Gallery intervention in three different low socio-economic classrooms indicated how the increased focus on learning over behaviour generated more positive responses to learning from the students, that the combined student voice in the data from across the three contexts communicated messages of high achievement, capability, and shared control, and that across each context, the students were developing emotional connections to the Gallery.

Focus on Learning Not Behaviour

The research occurred in educational settings that have traditionally been perceived and labelled 'challenging', for example, housing estates and urban multicultural suburbs. The pedagogical focus for learners in these contexts can often default to instruction in the basics and, as such, many students are often denied creative and artistic pedagogical practices due to the perceived potential for challenging behaviour (Munns et al., 2013;

Munns, 2021). The group-focused and playful nature of the pedagogy appeared to influence solidarity within each class group. This unity fuelled a growing 'insider' student concept and supported an emerging classroom atmosphere that all learners were included and that their involvement was meaningful.

The data highlighted that an important point for analysis was that the Gallery aligned with the notion that 'learning trumps behaviour' (Munns et al., 2013). The Gallery tasks, centred on creative, collaborative, and artistic forms of expression, which helped to build a focus on enjoyable and intellectually stimulating learning (Winchester, 2021). In each context, there was a key aim to work towards developing a culture of belonging. In this sense, '... individual students who are "outside" the accepted patterns of learning and behaviour are embraced and encouraged to join the classroom community' (Munns et al., 2013, p. 50). There were many instances when students who could be traditionally positioned as low-academic and/or having behavioural problems were showing more engaged learning and achieving Gallery outcomes at high levels. Apart from minor behavioural disruptions early in each school context, the pedagogical conditions of the Galleries allowed students to become 'insiders' in their classrooms and in each classroom context, a growing culture of belonging was strengthened (Allen et al., 2018).

Engaging Messages

An important finding across all sites was that the students began to speak in the language of engagement and that the message systems present in the data from each Gallery encouraged the learners to begin to identify as 'insiders' in their classrooms. Positive student self-concepts evolved over time, and it was a commonality that each group of students, by the end of the program, had strong involvement in their classroom learning. This appeared to be fostered by many factors, most significantly including high expectations of all students, the use of high affective, high operative and high cognitive tasks, student collaboration, inclusive class discussions, developing links to the wider school community and creating an environment for students to have a say in their own learning. These findings are consistent with Winchester (2021) and the Fair Go Program (FGP, 2013) that highlighted when students receive engaging messages there is a greater potential for them to value their learning and to develop a more enduring relationship with schooling (Munns et al., 2013).

The recurring outcome of these messages in each context, indicated that the students saw themselves as active participants in the learning of the Gallery. Their active involvement included not only their participation in the physical activities but their voice in class discussions and the shared control they held in classroom processes, and perhaps, most significantly, in the Exhibition.

Emotional Connection to Learning

An important outcome of the Gallery was that the students' emotional connection to the topics of study appeared to increase. One key aim was to prompt students to think and feel empathically within their topics of study. The students were given opportunities in each Gallery, through artistic and creative pedagogy, to empathically connect to the curriculum focus. The students began to express this through movement, drama, music, and through written and verbal forms. They also showed an increased understanding of the emotion within their topics and their ability to make sense of the actions or thoughts of the characters from their core texts. In approaching the Exhibitions, students expressed a desire to send empathic messages to an audience. Such evidence brought to light the more positive perceptions that the students held about themselves as valuable and capable learners with important knowledge to share.

In each instance the Exhibition presentation to the school community, as a culmination and celebration of the learning that had occurred throughout the Gallery program, demonstrated that each class was emotionally connected to their learning. This was not only evident in the responses in the classroom observation data but also in the students' expressions of enjoyment of the process, as evidenced in their Gallery reflections, further indicating that the students viewed their work as important, relevant, and meaningful.

Conclusion

The heart of the Gallery emerged, over time, to become the compassionate and emotional expressions of the students during their experiences. The concept of 'wise humanising creativity' and (posthumanising) creativity (Chappell, 2018), surfaced at the intersection of the research foci of student engagement, socio-emotional learning, arts-based pedagogy, and creativity. Humanising creativity appealed to a more communal and ethical version of creativity through using inherently human practices such as group work, shared responsibility, a focus on learning, shared goals, reflective practice, and, ultimately, a focus on 'big ideas' of human importance.

The Exhibition became a rich expression of artistic learning and not a fanciful artistic 'show'. It allowed these disadvantaged students to accentuate their feeling of ownership as part of the insider classroom mentality theorised in this study. For this reason, it was seen less as a 'product' of learning and more of an invitation to audience into the 'process' of the Gallery learning. As an example, one of the Exhibitions in one context culminated with the students not only expressing their emotional response to the experiences of those of The Stolen Generation, but also led them to relate these stories with their own family's history and migration stories of displacement, sorrow, and injustices.

The pedagogical model for the enactment of artistic learning in this research did not consider affective feeling and cognitive demands as binary opposites but argued for their interdependence and interaction as vital to authentic learning. Thus, the study points to how artistic pedagogy can be adopted with student engagement as one of the thematic drivers towards authentic learning.

The arts-based learning was put forward as a central pedagogical tool to intellectually stimulate, deploy high expectations, and enact a supportive classroom environment that aimed to emulate insider classroom feelings for students who were disadvantaged and who frequently found difficulty engaging in the school curriculum. In the development of the arts-based programs, New South Wales Education Standards Authority curriculum and syllabus documents were used to ensure that students were addressing the mandatory content and outcomes. The arts-based pedagogy deployed within the lessons appeared to provide a conduit to help students to think critically and meaningfully about human experiences and big ideas within the syllabus. By focussing more on pedagogy through the medium of art, this ameliorated behavioural issues, and increased student engagement, learning, their emotional health, and empathy with human issues. Many schools currently struggle with ways to include learners with more complex behavioural needs. This insight provides an opportunity for schools and systems to examine the effectiveness of their current practices to engage these students and to consider less prominence on behavioural modification programs, and greater emphasis on an alternative approach such as an arts-based pedagogy.

References

Allen, K., Kern, M. L., Vella-Brodrick, D., Hattie, J., & Waters, L. (2018). What schools need to know about fostering school belonging: A meta-analysis. *Educational Psychology Review, 30,* 1–34.

Almqvist, C. F., & Vist, T. (2019). Editorial special issue on arts-based research: Arts-based research in European arts education: Philosophical, ontological and epistemological introductions. *European Journal of Philosophy in Arts Education,* 4(01), 4–26.

Arthur, L., & Hertzberg, M. (2013) Culturally responsive pedagogical practices. In G. Munns, W. Sawyer, & B. Cole(Eds), *Exemplary teachers of students in poverty* (1st edn). Routledge. <https://doi.org/10.4324/9780203076408>.

Baldacchino, J. (2019). A brief critical historical analysis of neoliberalism in education. In S. Chitpin & Portelli, J. P. (Eds), *Confronting educational policy in neoliberal times: International perspectives* (pp. 11–24). Routledge.

Barone, T., & Eisner, E. W. (2012). *Arts based research.* Sage.

Brydon-Miller, M., Greenwood, D., & Maguire, P. (2003). Why action research? *Action Research*, *1*(1), 9–28.
Burnard, P., & Loughrey, M. (2021). Creativities of change in primary education. In P. Burnard & Loughrey, M. (Eds), *Sculpting new creativities in primary education* (pp. 3–25). Routledge.
Chappell, K. (2018). From wise humanising creativity to (posthumanising) creativity. In K. Snepvangers, P. Thomson, P. & A Harris (Eds), *Creativity policy, partnerships and practice in education* (pp. 279–306).
Craft, A. (2015). Possibility thinking. In *The Routledge international handbook of research on teaching thinking* (pp. 346–375). Springer Link.
Delamont, S. (2002). *Fieldwork in educational settings: Methods, pitfalls and perspectives*. Psychology Press.
Dewey, J. (1938). *Experience and education*. New York: Macmillan Company.
Egan, K. (2019). Honouring the role of narrative and metaphor in education. In M. Hanne & A. Kaal (Eds), *Narrative and metaphor in education: Looking both ways* (pp. 21–31). Routledge.
Fair Go Team. (2006). *School is for me: Pathways to student engagement*. Sydney: NSW Department of Education and Training.
Forlin, C., & Cooper, P. (2013). Student behavior and emotional challenges for teachers and parents in Hong Kong. *British Journal of Special Education*, *40*(2), 58–64.
Garrett, R., & MacGill, B. (2021). Fostering inclusion in school through creative and body-based learning. *International Journal of Inclusive Education*, *25*(11), 1221–1235.
Halverson, E., & Sawyer, K. (2022). Learning in and through the arts. *Journal of the Learning Sciences*, *31*(1), 1–13.
Hayes, D., Mills, M., Christie, P., & Lingard, B. (2006). *Teachers & schooling making a difference: Productive pedagogies, assessment and performance (Studies in education)*. Allen & Unwin.
Hernandez, I. A., Silverman, D. M., & Destin, M. (2021). From deficit to benefit: Highlighting lower-SES students' background-specific strengths reinforces their academic persistence. *Journal of Experimental Social Psychology*, *92*, 104080.
Lingard, B. (2013). *Politics, policies and pedagogies in education: The selected works of Bob Lingard*. Retrieved from <http://www.eblib.com>
Munns, G. (2004). *A sense of wonder: Student engagement in low SES school communities*. Paper presented at the Australian Association for Research Annual Conference, Melbourne, Australia, December 2004.
Munns, G. (2021). All about MeE: The Fair Go Program's student engagement framework. *Journal of Professional Learning*, *13*, 3–7.

Munns, G., & Sawyer, W. (2013). Student engagement: The research methodology and the theory. In G. Munns, W. Sawyer, & B. Cole (Eds), *Exemplary teachers of students in poverty* (pp. 14–32). Routledge.

Munns, G., Hatton, C., & Gilbert, S. (2013). Teaching in low socio-economic status communities. In G. Munns, W. Sawyer, & B. Cole (Eds), *Exemplary teachers of students in poverty* (pp. 33–46). Routledge.

NSW Premier and Cabinet. (2013). *Western Sydney demographics*. Retrieved from <http://www.westernsydney.nsw.gov.au/about-western-sydney/demographics/>

Orlando, J., & Sawyer, W. (2013). A fair go in education. In G. Munns, W. Sawyer, & B. Cole (Eds), *Exemplary teachers of students in poverty* (pp. 1–13). Routledge.

Riddle, S., Howell, A., McGregor, G., & Mills, M. (2021). Student engagement in schools serving marginalised communities. *International Journal of Inclusive Education, 28*(6) 1–16.

Ritchhart, R., Church, M., & Morrison, K. (2011). *Making thinking visible: How to promote engagement, understanding, and independence for all learners*. Wiley.

Sawyer, W., & Munns, G. (2019). Alternative messages of hope: Pedagogies, consensus and a fairer go. In *Confronting educational policy in neoliberal times* (1st edn, pp. 145–160). Routledge. <https://doi.org/10.4324/9781315149875-11>.

Sawyer, W., Munns, G., Zammit, K., Attard, C., Vass, E., & Hatton, C. (2018). *Engaging schooling: Developing exemplary education for students in poverty*. Routledge.

Siburian, J., Corebima, A. D., & Saptasari, M. (2019). The correlation between critical and creative thinking skills on cognitive learning results. *Eurasian Journal of Educational Research, 19*(81), 99–114.

Winchester, K. (2021). 'We are not just some kids': The gallery as a classroom space for student engagement. *Journal of Professional Learning, 13*, 30–38.

COLLEEN MCLAUGHLIN

12 Looking the Wrong Way

Introduction

The chapter explores a vital current issue in education, namely the lack of attendance and inclusion in school and how this is related to the mental health of students. The numbers of those missing school have now reached levels unknown in the British education system: a quarter of children miss significant amounts of education. This chapter explores the factors contributing to this, particularly the socio-political environment, and argues it is a parallel situation to that of the rise in exclusions in 2000 with similar serious consequences. It then discusses a current matter of concern interlinked with the exclusion-attendance issue, namely the mental health of children and young people and how schools may promote their students' mental health. Both issues were significant areas of work for Paul Cooper. The work that he and a team undertook on exclusions, reported in *Positive Alternatives to School* was awarded the TES Academic Book of the Year prize, while his contribution to mental health was substantial and had many facets, particularly his work on nurture groups, ADHD, psycho-social and biological interactions, and interventions for students with social, emotional and behaviour difficulties.

Background

'One day Nasrudin was outside his house. He was on his hands and knees frantically searching for something under a lamp post when his friend passed by and asked him what he was looking for. 'My key,' he said to his friend, 'I lost the key to my house.'

His friend being a nice person also got down on his hands and knees and tried to help him look. Some time passed. Eventually it was so dark they could barely see each other, when his friend asked him where he had lost his key. 'I lost it inside the house', Nasrudin replied. 'If you lost your key inside the house,' his friend asked him very confused, 'then why are we looking for it outside?' 'Because.' Nasrudin said with a gleam in his eyes, 'this is where the light is.' (Iyer, 2014)

In this chapter I argue that we may be looking in the wrong place for strategies to bring to the current issue of exclusion from school, as we did in 1996. In that year Paul Cooper and myself were in a team at the then School of Education, University of Cambridge that undertook the PASE project (Cooper et al., 2000) – an examination of positive alternatives to school exclusion. It was driven by a 400% rise in the annual rate of permanent exclusion from school between 1991 and 1996. The debates and possible reasons for this that were shared at the time focused upon unruly pupils and the need for teachers to be protected from these young people by establishing separate provision. This was strongly advocated by a union at the time. It located the problem in the children. Our knowledge of schools and teachers suggested to us that exclusion and ascribing the problem to the students was not an acceptable way forward. We also knew of schools that were not excluding any pupils at all. We invite/d schools to join us if they were interested in researching how a school staff could develop alternative inclusive practices and use existing research and thinking to inform the development of such practices, something that had not occurred before.

Our thinking was informed by other researchers' work (Hayden, 1997; Kinder et al., 1999; Parsons, 1999; Stirling, 1996) which had made a strong case for the link between educational policy, rates of exclusion and the disproportionate exclusion of students with special educational needs. At the time of this research, there was much evidence of the changed practice in the education system because of the 1988 Education Reform Act, a piece of legislation that established a new curriculum; accountability mechanisms such as Ofsted; and a market view of the education system including competition between schools. We argued that there was a link between the policy environment and the important, in this case negative, impact on young peoples' lives, opportunities and educational outcomes. There was much discussion of the move to *standards of education,* and some argued that the outcome of seeking for standards had created standardisation rather than high standards for all (Hayden, 1997). Ball (1993, p. 108) argued that these changes had created a 'new value context' which significantly impacted upon how educators perceived and constructed their responsibilities for appropriate provision for vulnerable children or those with emotional and behavioural difficulties. Thus, a central question is raised with reference to the inclusion of different groups and the nature of the common school: Who is the school for and what are its common purposes?

Inclusion in School

The inclusion of all children in schooling is a human right. Our concern in the PASE project (Cooper et al., 2000) was with the damage done to young people by exclusion from school and the frequent consequence of exclusion from society as a result 'coupled with a recognition that exclusionary practice effectively debars students from their moral entitlement to mainstream educational services' (Cooper et al., 2000, p. 5). This concern has become more complex due to even further changes in our society and in access to education in the UK, in particular the current issues of the continuing rise in exclusion rates and the new problem of 'ghost children'.

Rising Exclusions for Certain Groups

Using official Government data, NASEN (2022) noted that although 'permanent exclusions have reduced ... just under 4,000 children were permanently excluded [in 2020–21] ... remembering that most children were not in education settings at the time due to the pandemic. Regarding suspensions, the number rose considerably by over 40,000 to a total of over 350,000 suspensions'. A deeper examination of the headline figures shows that students of the following classifications had much higher rates of suspension and exclusion in comparison to their peers.

- The rate of suspension and exclusion amongst students identified as Free School Meals (FSM) was *four times higher* than that of their peers.
- Students with an EHC [education, health and care] plan had a rate of suspension and exclusion that was *double* of their peers.
- Students identified as needing SEN support had a rate of suspension and exclusion *five times higher* than that of their peers.
- The rate of suspension and exclusion amongst Roma students was *six times higher* than that of their peers.
- The permanent exclusion rates of mixed White and Black Caribbean were *four times higher* than those of their peers.
- The exclusion rate of students from the Northeast of England was four times higher than the South East. (NASEN, 2022).

The continuous rise in exclusion and suspension suggests we have not yet fully addressed this problem and since as Ball (1993) noted, the changed 'value context' of the time is built through policy making and actions, there are questions which need to be asked about this relationship now.

Ghost Children

The phrase 'ghost children' applies to students not at their desks more than 50% of the time. A recent report by the Centre for Social Justice (2023) found that the number of severely absent, 'ghost children' rose from 93,000 in the autumn of 2020 to 140,000 in the summer of 2022. Obviously, the arrangements for education during this period had a major impact on these figures – schools were closed much of the time, there was online learning and high anxiety about the epidemic. However, the number of severely absent children has continued and is now at an all-time high. 'This represents a rise of 134% since the last term before the pandemic, Autumn 2019. It is the equivalent of 137 entire schools where the children are mostly missing lessons.' (Centre for Social Justice, 2023). In addition, one in fifty children are regularly skipping lessons despite remaining on class rolls. Absenteeism rates are highest in the most disadvantaged areas and more than 110,000 of these students (78% of the total severely absent children) are from state-funded secondary schools. The report states that the level of absenteeism across all secondary schools is equivalent to every class losing a student.

Moreover, nearly two million children are persistently absent from school (absent more than 10% of the time). More than a quarter of children are missing classes on a regular basis and the rate of persistent absence is double the rate of persistent absence pre-pandemic. The report exposes the many reasons children are missing school including increased anxiety and mental health problems, unmet special educational needs/disabilities, and issues at home. 'The stark fact is that more than a quarter of children are missing school at a significant level' (Centre for Social Justice, 2023).

What might be the implications of this data? First the Covid pandemic clearly presented very challenging circumstances that have had major impacts on all aspects of society. However, the impact has not been equally felt on all students alike. There has been an amplification of the trend that the disadvantaged are more at risk. In the conclusion to *Positive Alternative to Exclusion* (Cooper et al., 2000, p. 186) we raised the question of what makes a difference to inclusion or exclusion in schools, and we determined that, '*Everything* makes a difference. Every act of meaning making, as students and staff process their school experience, contributes in some to how they respond to that experience'. It would appear that there is a lack of congruence between the goals and aspirations of staff, students, parents and policy makers as a significant percentage of students have not returned to school. Is it because they do not feel they fit or belong or that school is not relevant to their present situation? This is not to undermine or question the good intentions of school actors but rather to suggest that the idea of the common school or the comprehensive school is in need of tough interrogation. To parody the words of George Orwell in 1945, it seems some animals fit more easily than others into the school of today.

Secondly, if we accept that there is a relationship between the policy environment and what is occurring in practice then we need to examine that relationship and look at the framework adopted to explain the problems. I have presented earlier on how that was in the year 2000. Today we still see an absence of examining the systemic contribution when we examine problems in schooling. There is a clear trend that certain students do not progress, succeed as well or even attend in some cases. These are the disadvantaged students and those who exhibit difference. We have also lived through a time of rising inequality and increased poverty in the UK. Clearly this is relevant and is a debate in itself, but equality matters in education, and we seem to have run out of new approaches in addressing this issue. In a comprehensive examination of schools today, Tim Brighouse and Mick Waters (2021, p. 574) concluded that, 'The school system in England needs consensus about its purpose'. The recent figures around exclusion and attendance support this conclusion and show that the current state of affairs is not sustainable if we are to meet the needs of all students as is their human right. Like Nasrudin, we may need to look elsewhere for the key to this problem, beyond the obvious and easy places.

Mental Health and Schools

Are there parallels between the debate about exclusion rates and non-attendance at school and those about the mental ill-health amongst our young people? The Covid epidemic was a powerful factor in struggles with mental health for adults and children alike and a UK State of the Nation report into young people's mental health summarised their enquiry thus:

> Overall, the findings presented in this report suggest an inconsistent recovery of children and young people's wellbeing and mental health towards pre-pandemic levels by the end of the 2021/22 academic year. While annual trends indicated that children and young people's subjective happiness and life satisfaction appears to have recovered to pre-pandemic levels by 2022 (The Children's Society, 2022), some measures, such as anxiousness among primary and secondary age pupils (DfE, 2002a, 2022b), and loneliness (DfE, 2022c) and mental health among older young people (NHS Digital, 2022), may have worsened further. However, it is not clear from these data why this might be the case. In addition, the percentage of those reporting low happiness with their health appears to have increased in recent years (The Children's Society, 2015, 2016, 2017, 2018, 2019, 2020, 2021, 2022) and eating problems remain at elevated levels compared to before the COVID-19 pandemic (NHS Digital, 2022).

> While a range of individual and societal factors may have contributed to this, the current data do not allow us to make strong claims about the main causes of these trends. (DFE, 2023, p. 17)

Some of the above conclusions mirror other data on exclusions. There is a tendency for different groups and concerns to be disproportionately represented. One of the key elements is poverty. The concerns in the DFE study (2023, p. 19). were 'about household finances' with around a third of parents and carers reporting that they had struggled with school costs' and around one in five of 7- to 16-year-olds and one in ten of 17- to 22-year-olds reported that their household had experienced a reduction in income in the previous twelve months (NHS Digital, 2022), suggesting worsening of household finances for some families in the previous year. Finance and annual household income affected time spent outside and a connection to nature and engagement in physical activity. Inequality was a recurrent theme as well as race and gender. The opportunities to spend time outside varied between white children and those from ethnic minorities; between those with and without a disability and between genders.

Mental Health, School and Young People

Gray et al. (2011) investigated a sub theme of the Nuffield study of 'changed adolescence': the evidence on the relationship between school experience and mental health outcomes. Their conclusions affirmed, as others had before, that schools were very important indeed in young people's development and have been described as second only to families in their impact on the wellbeing of young people. As Rutter (1991, p. 9) wrote, 'Schooling does matter greatly. Moreover, the benefits can be surprisingly long lasting ... Schools are about social experiences as well as scholastic learning.' Rutter also showed how many of the school factors became protective later on in life. Schools could be nurturing environments and could play a significantly positive role in shaping mental health in young people. It is an ecological view of young people and their development:

> Human beings create the environments that shape the course of human development. Their actions influence the multiple physical and cultural tiers of the ecology that shapes them, and this agency makes humans – for better or for worse – active producers of their own development. (Bronfenbrenner, 2005, p. xxvii).

The Nuffield review (2012) identified a range of school factors that related to young people's sense of wellbeing. These included relationships with teachers, relationships with peers and general satisfaction with the educational experience. All of these contribute to greater feelings of 'school connectedness'. A sense of detachment from school grows as adolescents get older and young people with special educational needs are identified as especially vulnerable here. Gustafson et al. (2010, p. 161) argued that early school failure 'can cause marked internalizing and externalizing mental health problem', and they too pointed out that relations with peers and teachers could serve as a protective factor. The Gray study (2011, p. 106) concluded that, 'the most important factor affecting young people's well-being relates to the cultures of support their schools develop and sustain'.

Where to Look and at What

Recent data suggests that there has been an increase in mental health difficulties amongst young people. It had steadied in its rise but in the last five years it has risen again. One in six children/adolescents experience serious mental health problems and UK rates of depression, anxiety, self-harm, substance misuse, suicide are among the highest economically well off countries (Good Childhood Report, 2020a; OECD, 2021). 'Young people have reported much higher levels of anxiety and depression since the onset of the COVID-19 pandemic compared with the general adult population, widening existing differences' (OECD, 2021). Physical health, substance misuse, homelessness, criminality and suicidality are actually rising.

When looking for strategies and approaches that schools could use to contribute to a reduction in these social, emotional and behavioural problems, the national response has been first to focus on services for individuals. The Children's Society (2022b) argues for a faster rollout of mental health support teams in schools. They also argue for early support hubs in every community which should work with mental health teams, in order to stop young people having to wait for help. The role of the school has been constructed as 'identifying mental health needs at an early stage, referring young people to specialist support and working jointly with others to support young people experiencing problems' (DHSE & DfE, 2017, p. 10). It is a health or medical model which emphasises diagnosis and treatment; this is the approach taken with children with SEND many decades ago. This is to suggest that the most important area of intervention is with the individual. It is self-evident that we should help individuals and should relieve their distress but there are other strategies for schools to develop good mental health in young people.

The second approach is a more developmental or educational one, that is to focus upon specialist educational programmes such as mindfulness, anxiety management or resilience developing strategies. This approach is one that aims to remedy a particular issue by intervening with a group through education. It is using counselling or psychological knowledge in an educative rather than a solely remedial way.

While such individual and educational strategies are useful, and are important levels and arenas of work, such an approach ignores the contribution of the environment to the problem. There is mounting evidence that the policy and practice environment and the psychosocial environment of young people are a major influence and contribute to the mental health of young people. There has been a thread of significant research studies since the 1980s and the beginning of the 'schools make a difference' movement. These studies look at the specific factors in schools and in the social environments of young people that may be underlying the mental health difficulties and work on changing them. This is to work on the policy and practice and requires work in other arenas. This way of seeing and framing requires us, as Nasrudin's friend suggested, to look for where we lost our 'key'. Rutter's research in the early 1990s seems quite prophetic (Rutter, 1991). He argued strongly that we must treat schools as nurturing environments and that seeing the long-term impact of school experiences was vital. In commenting that we are focusing on the wrong questions, he wrote, 'to a very considerable extent how we act serves to shape and select later environments. Environments do not come randomly; we do things that *influence the experiences that we have* (my italics). In other words, the question of whether early experiences have effects that are independent of later experiences is artificial and misleading because it ignores the very important fact that later environments in reality are determined in part, often large part, by earlier experiences' (Rutter 1991, p. 6). This is very similar to the conclusion of the *Positive Alternatives to Exclusion* project (Cooper et al., 2000), that is, when we ask what matters, everything matters.

Rutter (1991) identified key outcomes that aid young people's development (raised self-efficacy and self-esteem along with skills that enhance task-orientation and persistence), but he was also concerned with wider educational practices and policy. 'The message is that, in itself, the acquisition of facts is *not* a sensible sufficient goal for schools. ... the goals of schooling must include social features as well as the transmission of information. In years gone by, educationalists have debated whether *either* a task-oriented, nose-to-the-grindstone approach *or* an emotionally supportive approach designed to make children want to be at school and enjoy their learning was better. The choice is artificial and misleading... positive school experiences made it more likely that young people would exert planning in their lives ...' (Rutter, 1991, p. 7). The Good Childhood Report (2022a, p. 32) underlined the validity of these concerns: 'More children (aged 10–17) are unhappy with school than with the other aspects of life they are asked about ... We found that happiness with school and schoolwork declines significantly with age and is far lower among children in lower income households' and those with disability.

The import of social disconnectedness in school experience has come to the fore in another recent research. In a 2021 a large-scale study of 29,086 high school students in Denmark highlighted the role of the school as a connecting socially focused organisation: 'Our results add to a large evidence-base suggesting that mental health problems among adolescents may be prevented by promoting social connectedness at school ... fostering social connectedness at school may prevent loneliness' (Santini et al., 2021, p. 1). This and other studies point to the importance of the wider social goals for education and for them to drive practice in a much stronger way than is currently evident. This merits exploring key practices such as pedagogical approaches, assessment and feedback processes, which have a deep effect on young people' sense of self and significance.

Carol Dweck and her body of research on mindsets and young people have advocated for a paradigm shift. She has shown the role of young people's mindsets in 'their seeking of challenges and their thriving amid setbacks' (Yeager & Dweck, 2023, p. 79). By mindset she means, 'beliefs about the nature of working of human attributes such as intelligence or personality'. She distinguishes between two types of mindsets: fixed and growth. A growth mindset refers to the 'belief that change and growth are possible under the right conditions; on the other hand, in a fixed mindset "challenges and setbacks risk judgement of low (permanent) ability"' (Yeager & Dweck, 2023, p. 79). Space precludes a full exposition of these two mindsets, but they are affected by school practices and frameworks such as adoption of a normality distribution approach to ability, feedback practices, fixed educational practices, and an emphasis on right answers rather than experimentation and flexible outcomes. The evidence suggests that students who are encouraged to develop a fixed mindset are at risk of depression, developing learned helplessness and becoming preoccupied with saving face rather than being open to 'failure' and experimentation (Dweck, 2000).

The recent emphasis on the outcomes of tests, a focus on knowledge retention and accountability is the ideal ground for the development of a fixed mindset – the opposite of the resilience and persistence necessary to engage with the complexities of the modern world. Yeager and Dweck (2023) have engaged in designing two scalable, manageable educational interventions (The National Study of Learning Mindsets) that involved a digital programme subject to a random control design testing. They conducted their study which involved educating young people about the plasticity of the brain and then in a later phase about mindsets and how they develop. They targeted depressed and anxious youth and with impressive results. 'Across three randomized controlled double-blind trials totalling 598 9th grade students, the growth mindset programme led to a 36% relative reduction in the onset of clinically significant symptoms of depression over the 9-month school year' (Yeager & Dweck, 2023, p. 80).

Conclusion

In this chapter, we have seen the benefits of engaging with education as a tool that aims for social and emotional impact, an education that is engaging, encourages agency, sense of belonging, connection and the formation of significant relationships. Undertaking this goal has implications for *everything* in school – assessment, sought after outcomes, content, autonomy, classroom practices and organisation, pedagogy, and the language used in feedback. This is what forms the bedrock of good mental health for young people. We need also to address the non-attendance and exclusion rises which have resulted in nearly 20% of the school population being away from school. Schools will have to evolve and look back at the dark places they have not looked yet. Education policy makers have spent too much time looking for the key under the lamplight. The lack of autonomy for schools, a rigid inspection framework and regime have inadvertently made a significant contribution to the rise in mental health issues amongst young people. We now know enough from research to enable schools and their practices to contribute powerfully to the betterment of young people though creating enabling environments and practices. It involves a proactive approach where we aim to construct nurturing environments, ones where we examine all we do to see if it makes a contribution to good mental health or not. This would involve changing educational and social practices in school such as assessment models, focusing on knowledge acquisition as the only goal of education, and constraining schools in what they can do in responding to the young people in their care.

References

Ball, S. (1993). Education policy, power relations and teachers' work. *British Journal of Educational Studies, 42*(2), 106–121.

Brighouse, T., & Waters, M. (2021). *About our schools: Improving on previous best.* Crown House Publishing.

Bronfenbrenner, U. (Ed.). (2005). *Making human beings human: Bioecological perspectives on human development*. Sage.

Centre for Social Justice. (2023). *Lost and not found: How severe absence became endemic in England's schools*. <www.centreforsocialjustice.org.uk>.

The Children's Society. (2015). *The good childhood report 2015*. <https://www.basw.co.uk/system/files/resources/basw_14829-10_0.pdf>.

The Children's Society. (2016). *The good childhood report 2016*. <https://www.basw.co.uk/system/files/resources/basw_94045-10_0.pdf>.

The Children's Society. (2017). *The good childhood report 2017*. <https://www.basw.co.uk/system/files/resources/basw_53118-7_0.pdf>.

The Children's Society. (2018). *The good childhood report 2018*. <https://www.basw.co.uk/system/files/resources/thegood_childhood_report_20 18_0.pdf>.

The Children's Society. (2019). *The good childhood report 2019*. <https://saphna.co/wp-content/uploads/2019/11/the_good_childhood_report_2019.pdf>.

The Children's Society. (2020). *The good childhood report 2020*. <https://www.childrenssociety.org.uk/sites/default/files/2020-11/Good-Childhood-Report-2020.pdf>.

The Children's Society. (2021). *The good childhood report 2021*. <https://www.childrenssociety.org.uk/information/professionals/resources/good-childhood-report-2021>.

The Children's Society. (2022a). *The good childhood report 2022*. <https://www.childrenssociety.org.uk/information/professionals/resources/good-childhood-report-2022>.

The Children's Society. (2022b). *The good childhood report 2022: Summary and recommendations*. The Children's Society.

Cooper, P., Drummond, M. J., Hart, S., Lovey, J., & McLaughlin, C. (2000). *Positive alternatives to exclusion*. Routledge.

Department for Education Research report. (2023). *State of the nation 2022: Children and young people's wellbeing*. Department for Education.

DfE. (2022a). *Parent, pupil and learner panel omnibus surveys for 2021 to 2022*. Retrieved from <https://www.gov.uk/government/publications/parent-pupil-and-learner-panel-omnibus-surveys-for-2021-to-2022>.

DfE. (2022b). *Parent, pupil and learner panel – June wave*. Retrieved from <www.assets.publishing.service.gov.uk/media/639219408fa8f53baa1f3f5f/PPLP_report_rw4_june.pdf>.

DfE. (2022c). *Parent, pupil and learner panel – May wave*. Retrieved from <www.assets.publishing.service.gov.uk/media/63921930e90e0766390d925c/PPLP_report_rw3_may.pdf>.

DHSS and DFE. (2017). *Transforming children and young people's mental health provision: A green paper*. Crown Publications.

Dweck, C. S. (2000). *Self-theories: Their role in motivation, personality, and development.* Psychology Press.

Gray, J., Galton, M., McLaughlin, C., Clark, B., & Symonds, J. (2011). *The supportive school – wellbeing and the young adolescent.* Cambridge Scholars Publishing.

Gustafsson, J., Westling, M. A., Åkerman, B. A., Eriksson, C., Eriksson, L., Fischbein, S., ... Persson, R. S. (2010). *School, learning and mental health a systematic review.* The Health Committee, Royal Swedish Academy of Sciences.

Hamblin, D. H. (1978). *The teacher and counselling.* Basil Blackwell.

Hayden, C. (1997). *Children excluded from primary school: Debates, evidence, responses.* Open University Press.

Iyer, D. S. 'The Darkness Is the Key'. (2014). *Psychology Today* online. Retrieved from <https://www.psychologytoday.com/us/blog/life-liberty-and-the-pursuit-insight/201403/the-darkness-is-the-key>.

Kinder, K., Jendall, S., Downing, D., Atkinson, M., & Hogarth, S. (1999). *Raising behaviour 2: Nil exclusion? Policy and practice.* National Foundation for Educational Research.

NASEN (National Association of Special Educational Needs). (2022). *Data on permanent exclusions and suspensions reveals rates for children with SEN is five times higher.* Retrieved from <https://nasen.org.uk/news/data-permanent-exclusions-and-suspensions-reveals-rates-children-sen-five-times-higher>.

NHS Digital. (2022). *Mental health of children and young people in England 2022 – wave 3 follow up to the 2017 survey.* Retrieved from <https://digital.nhs.uk/data-and-information/publications/statistical/mental-health-of-children-and-young-people-in-england/2022-follow-up-to-the-2017-survey>.

Nuffield Foundation. (2012). *Social trends and mental health: Introducing the main findings.* Nuffield Foundation.

OECD. (2021). *Fitter minds, fitter jobs: From awareness to change in integrated mental health, skills and work policies, mental health and work.* OECD Publishing. <https://doi.org/10.1787/0815dof-en>.

Orwell, G. (1945). *Animal farm.* Penguin.

Parsons, C. (1999). *Education, exclusion and citizenship.* Routledge.

Rutter, M. (1991). Pathways to and from childhood to adult life: The role of schooling. *Pastoral Care in Education, 9*(3), 3–10. <https://doi.org/10.3389/fnbeh.2021.632906>.

Stirling, M. (1996). Government policy and disadvantaged children. In E. Blythe & J. Milner (Eds), *Exclusion from school: Inter-professional issues for policy and practice* (pp. 53–61). Routledge.

Yeager, D., & Dweck, C. S. (2023). Mindsets and adolescent mental health. *Nature Mental Health, 1,* 79–81.

MARIA POULOU

13 From Students 'without voices' to Students with ... 'low voices'

Introduction

The acknowledgement of students' voices and empowerment in inclusive education is evident in policy initiatives internationally. However there still exists the gap between educational policy and practice. Although studies on the perspectives of pupils with special educational needs have increased, very few studies focus on the voices of students identified as students with social, emotional and behavioural difficulties (SEBD). This chapter, taking Paul Cooper's (1989) work on residential EBD children's views as a starting point, aims to delineate research on SEBD students' voices in Greece within the spectrum of educational policy and research in Europe. Despite the advocacy of inclusive education in policy documents, in Greece there is still lack of attention on the voices of SEBD students. The constraints and the benefits of having students' voices heard are discussed, leading to the conclusion that the voiceless SEBD students in the past are still waiting for the opportunity to be heard.

Educational Policies and Practices on Students' Voices

The first chapter written for children's rights, and which showed the way for the recognition of inclusive education was the Warnock Report 1978 (Pappas et al., 2018). Following this report, an emphasis on students' rights was made with the United Nations Convention on the Rights of the Child in 1989, and the specific articles 12 and 13 focusing on students' views, the Salamanca statement (UNESCO, 1994), the United Nations Convention on the Rights of People with Disabilities (United Nations, 2006), and the Incheon Declaration (UNICEF, 2015). These documents legitimised student voice and started the discussion about the views of children and particularly the views of at-risk children which can challenge policymakers (Ainscow & Messiou, 2017).

Based on the already applied models of social welfare and education in other countries, in Greece there is evidence of improvement in the field of special education, with an increase in the number of inclusive classes (Pappas et al., 2018). Education Law 1143/81 was the first comprehensive law in the history of Special Education in Greece (Tafa & Manolitsis, 2003), which was however criticised because it marginalised Special Education from the Core of General Education. Education Law 1566/1985 was one of the most important laws in recent Greek education because it institutionalised special education for the first-time. During the 1980s and the 1990s, special education was provided mainly in special schools, while as from 2000 a policy of educational integration and the model of 'one school for all' has been advocated (Syriopoulou-Delli, 2010). The beginning of the twenty-first century can be characterised as the symbolic starting point for the Greek inclusive discourse, with the language of social inclusion being central in discussions of social policy (Zoniou-Sideri et al., 2006). In March 2000 another law (Law 2817/2000) emphasised the common educational needs of students with disabilities and not on the clinical dimensions of their disabilities. According to this law special schools should be limited only to children with severe and multiple disabilities, whereas students with Special Education Needs (SEN) were assigned to special centres (Centers of Diagnosis and Support) (Bablekou & Kazi, 2016). Therefore, the inclusion of students with SEN into the education system has started to improve and their accessibility to building and other facilities has made progress. The teaching staff also received more specialised education through the Special Education University Departments.

According to Education Law 3699/2008 (European Agency for Special Needs and Inclusive Education (2020), the state is obliged to provide special educational provision to all children who are recognised as eligible for additional support, at all levels of the education system. Specifically, pupils with disabilities and/or special educational needs (SEN) are described as having significant difficulties in learning for the whole or some period of their school life, due to sensory, intellectual or developmental problems, mental health and neuropsychological disorders that affect the process of their school adjustment and learning (Article 3). Low achievers and learners with learning disabilities that derive from external factors, such as linguistic or cultural diversity, are not considered to have a disability or SEN. Pupils with complex cognitive, emotional and social difficulties, delinquent behaviour resulting from abuse, parental neglect and abandonment or domestic violence, and pupils with one or more special intellectual skills and talents, are considered to have SEN.

Education Law 4368/2016 (Article 82) (GG 21 A/2016) redefined the objectives of inclusion classes to avoid learners being discriminated against by being pulled out of mainstream classes to attend inclusion classes. It stresses that the main aim of the inclusion classes is the full inclusion of children with special education needs and/or disabilities in the class environment. In this context, inclusive education is among the priorities of the Greek educational system. The Ministry delivers policies and initiatives aimed at constantly providing quality of education for all pupils, including those with disabilities and/or special educational needs. Teachers of inclusive classes support the pupils within the mainstream classroom, in cooperation with the class teachers. They differentiate activities and educational practices and adapt the educational material and the educational environment. One to one support is only exceptionally provided in a separate inclusion classroom. In this case, the main target of the teaching intervention is the prospective full inclusion of the pupil in the mainstream class. In practical terms, a clear classification of students' SEN is missing, and the broad category of students with learning problems and/or social, emotional and behavioural difficulties is often used in practice.

Research on the Voices of Students with SEBD

Paul Cooper (1989) was one of the first to argue on the importance of studying students' own perspectives if we need to have a clear picture of what happens in schools. Listening to students' voice practically means respect and empowerment to promote positive experience in schools, which is the epitome of inclusion. Students' voice can be defined as the right to express their opinions, to access people who influence decisions, and to exercise active participation in educational decision-making process (Thomsen, 2011). Young people's education is an interactional process involving students and teachers, with participants' views, worries and perceptions given equal attention in a school climate of mutual respect and democracy. Listening to students' voices is reflected in the opportunities provided to students to participate meaningfully in improving their life in schools (Rudduck & McIntyre, 2007). Students are social agents (Rudduck & Flutter, 2000), and their authentic participation in educational decisions must be taken seriously (Shallcross et al., 2007). Sellman (2009) argues that it is important to differentiate between student empowerment initiatives that simply seek to give students opportunities to be heard, and genuine involvement. The idea of student voice encompasses a range of meaning and activities encouraging the involvement of young people in decision-making processes. This implies that students have the potential to bring about change in schools through their suggestions and active participation (Messiou et al., 2022).

International research on students' voices and empowerment in inclusive education has been increasing (Hartas & Geoff, 2011; Sellman, 2009). Using data from literature and policy documents from five European countries (Austria, Denmark, England, Portugal and Spain), Messiou et al. (2022) found that although the term 'student voice' is not used in policy documents in all five countries, there are numerous references to students' participation which signals the importance assigned to the idea of giving students the chance to be heard. Nonetheless, very few studies have focused on the voices of students with social emotional and behavioural difficulties (Davis, 2005; Flynn, 2013; Sellman, 2009). This group represents some of the most marginalised students in school and the least listened group compared to their peers (Cefai & Cooper, 2010; Herz & Haertel, 2016). Social, emotional and behavioural difficulties represent a unique category of difficulties among school students involving an interaction of educational issues, social policy, social welfare, mental health and criminal justice (Cooper, 2010).

Why the Voices of Students with SEBD Are Low?

There is evidence that students with SEBD provide valid and useful information on their experiences (Fielding & Bragg, 2003), and that their voice empowerment may minimise their difficulties experienced in schools (Cefai & Cooper, 2010). Nevertheless, they are the least liked group of students with educational needs (Cooper, 2001, 2006) with the least opportunities to express their perspective (Cefai & Spiteri Pizzuto, 2017).

One explanation is that these students might lack the confidence to express themselves or the possibility to articulate clearly, which links up with the problematic methodological approaches to address students' perspective in education (Kefallinou & Howes, 2002). SEBD phenomenon lies mainly on parents', teachers' and professionals' views of children experiences, rather the direct experiences of the child or young person themselves (de Leeuw et al., 2018; Georgiadi et al., 2020). Children and adolescents with disabilities are often left out of research because involving them can present extra methodological challenges for researchers since their individual characteristics are not always easy to aggregate into large data sets (Georgiadi et al., 2020). Research on students' voices therefore need to ensure alternative methods appropriate for students such as drawings, pictures, and storytelling amongst others (Cefai & Spiteri Pizzuto, 2017).

Many teachers perceive students with SEBD as objects of educational research (Christensen & James, 2008) and any effort for their empowerment is compromised by contexts determined by adults (Lewis & Burman, 2008). Adults may have little trust in students' capacity to express a valid opinion (Messiou & Hope, 2015) and sometimes they listen to learners in a manipulative way (Messiou & Hope, 2015), or in a collective voice (Cook-Sather, 2006) paying little attention to the individual needs of students with diverse experiences (Kefallinou & Howes, 2002). Moreover, the voices of students with SEBD remain silent because the students are viewed by educators as being the problem, rather than having the problem (Heary & Hennessy, 2005). This shapes how adults respond to students' behaviour and attribute blame for the behaviour (Caslin, 2019).

What Do Studies with Students with SEBD Say

Studies which have taken into consideration students' voices show different aspects of students' concerns. They all agree however, that students are considered important informants who need to be heard. Cooper (1989) initially investigated the perspectives of residential students with SEBD, with the aim to develop insights into the real-life experience of residential schools and to identify models of good practice. The concept of 're-signification' was introduced as the process to promote improvement in students' negative labelling effects and sense of identity. The study underlined the idea that to respond to learners' diversity and needs it is important to listen to students' perceptions and feelings.

Studies thereafter aimed to develop exploratory research strategies to strengthen the voice of children of children with SEBD, with a particular emphasis on involving the young people in the research process (O' Connor et al., 2011). Some of the themes which emerged from these studies on children's voices, included sense of victimization, exclusion and stigmatisation (Cefai & Cooper, 2010; de Leeuw et al., 2018), the impact of SEBD labels attached to them by others (Caslin, 2019), and their preferred approaches for resolving social problems (de Leeuw et al., 2018). Adolescents who were asked to assess the social factors related to their difficulties named negative family functioning, lack of academic motivation and absence of close friends, implying the need for a supportive social network for adolescents (Kapi et al., 2007). Mainstream students with learning problems or SEBD reported that their educational problems caused emotional reactions (feelings of anxiety, sadness, social participation and motivation problems (de Boer & Kuijper, 2021). Students also experience marginalisation and loneliness in the classrooms (Schwab, 2015) and difficulties in building relationships with peers (Krull et al., 2014). There are less studies however on students' perceptions on the evaluation of special schools' behaviour policy (Sellman, 2009), nurture classes (Cefai & Spiteri Pizzuto, 2017), the enablers and barriers to positive outcomes (Siobhan & Frederickson, 2013) or their own well-being (Georgiadi et al., 2020; Hall, 2010; Herz & Haertel, 2016).

Even though Greece has signed the Convention of the Rights of the Child (United Nations, 1989) and the Convention of the Rights of Persons with Disabilities (United Nations, 2006), nothing has been officially adopted on children's right to active participation in decision-making process in their education (Rouvali & Riga, 2021). Researchers have noted a lack of attention to the voices of vulnerable students, and stress that inclusion cannot be well understood without the representation of the views and experiences of these students based on the principles of fairness and equity (Kefallinou & Howes, 2002). Studies on students' perceptions in general education and in SEN are limited (Brouzos et al., 2015; Leontopoulou et al., 2011). Even more scarce are studies on the perspectives of students with SEBD, who are mainly educated in general education, reflecting the limited systematic evidence on the methods used to measure students' voices and the way these voices are portrayed in education (Palikara et al., 2018), or the reluctance of teachers and parents to recruit such students in research.

The limited number of studies In the Greek context reveals similarities with international findings. Avramidis and colleagues (2018) examined the views of students with SEN in inclusive settings and found that students with SEN in upper primary classes (9–11 years old) receive fewer nominations of peer acceptance, had fewer friends and fewer social interactions with classmates than their typically developing peers. Poulou and colleagues carried out various studies on the views of students with SEBD in relation to the predictors of their behaviour challenges, such as social information processes (Poulou & Bassett, 2018) and emotion knowledge (Poulou, 2019) in pre-school children, social skills (Poulou, 2014a) and teacher-student relationships (Poulou, 2017) in primary school, and personality characteristics (Poulou, 2010, 2013, 2014b) and sleep duration patterns (Poulou & Cooper, 2017) in secondary school. Adolescents' perceptions of their psychological needs (existence needs, peers relatedness needs, teacher relatedness needs and growth needs), mixed self-perceptions and well-being were also found to be potential predictors of students' school adjustment (Poulou & Norwich, 2020).

Why Do We Need to Make the Voices of Students with SEBD Louder?

Cooper (1993) advocated that we have a legal obligation to students, namely that not only should we take account students' perspectives, but as educators we have a moral obligation to help them to articulate their own views. This is the way towards understanding the effectiveness of provision and intervention at school. Secondly, the underlying principle shared by theoretical models is that SEBD are often embedded in the ways in which individuals perceive themselves and that SEBD change stems from the description and analysis of these perceptions. Thirdly, by taking into consideration students' perspective, we can evaluate the effectiveness of provision and intervention offered to students as well as be in a better position to identify models of good practice for SEBD interventions. Additional benefits of the inclusion of students' voices include improved academic, motivation and engagement and teachers' insights for improved practice (Sellman, 2009).

Conversely when students are ignored, they receive wrong messages of what effective teaching (Sellman, 2009) and close teacher-student relationships consist of. The lack of research on students' perspective also implies the reproduction of the medical model that SEBD are innate biological conditions (Herz & Haertel, 2016; Sellman, 2009) and students have no control on their behaviour. Understanding the complexities of the systemic influences in SEBD enables schools and those responsible in supporting students to carefully consider how conditions of adversity and disadvantage can be reinforced or negated by the system that they are a part of (Georgiadi et al., 2020).

When adequately addressed, students' voices offer strong evidence and highlight important issues around student identities (Kefallinou & Howes, 2002). Flynn (2013) summarised the major themes of related to the voices of students with SEBD as the importance of being heard, the perspective of difference, the relational care and school leadership. The consensus among these students is that they want to be respected whereas the negative teachers' attitudes contributed both to their negative opinions of themselves and to frustration and conflict with teachers (Flynn, 2013; Poulou, 2014a). Where teacher-student relationships are close, students' social and emotional skills and resilience are enhanced and students experience less difficulties (Poulou et al., 2022a, 2022b; Siobhan & Frederickson, 2013). Students' psychological adjustment can be addressed as long as their psychological needs of relatedness with teachers and peers are being met (Poulou & Norwich, 2020). Here is exactly where the power of student voice lies. Addressing students' psychological needs could help teachers and other school professionals to develop interventions to satisfy these needs. The satisfaction of students' needs may promote positive school outcomes and student's well-being. Research confirms students' involvement in planning, implementation and monitoring of change processes resulting in the improvement of students' educational outcomes (Siobhan & Frederickson, 2013). No matter how 'well-functioning' a system might be, if it is not perceived as such from a student point of view, it falls short (Kefallinou & Howes, 2002). This is particularly true of students with SEBD who may be more at risk of being excluded from the educational process (Cefai & Spiteri Pizzuto, 2017).

Conclusions

Capturing the voices of students with special educational needs has been recognised as a key element of policy initiatives internationally (United Nations, 2006). However, there still exists the gap between policy and practice both internationally and in Greece (Palikara et al., 2018). Cooper (1989) introduced research on the perspectives of students with SEBD and argued that effective schools are seen by their students as offering respite, relationships and opportunities (Cooper, 1993). Despite the growth of research including the views of young people, and the evidence that students with SEBD can provide valid and useful ideas in improving their school environment (Cefai & Cooper, 2010; O' Connor et al., 2011; Sellman, 2009), the voices of young students with SEBD continue to be among the least heard (Cefai & Cooper, 2010; Holdsworth & Blanchard, 2006). Research on presenting the voices of children is challenging since it requires appropriate methodology and care in eliciting and interpreting valid responses (Whitehurst, 2007). Student empowerment projects are more challenging to implement in provision for students with SEBD in mainstream schools and thus less frequently attempted (Sellman, 2009). Nevertheless, the adoption of a protagonist (student)-related research perspective is fundamental to the development of an inclusive learning environment for the benefit of all students.

An education system which promotes inclusive principles should encourage a culture of listening (Flynn, 2013). Students with SEBD have important messages to share regarding their educational experiences and can provide powerful insights that can help adults who work with them (Caslin, 2019). Supporting students with SEBD is demanding, but specific attention to their needs drives us towards the solution of their difficulties (Cooper, 2010). With the adoption of non-hierarchical lenses, educators and policy makers may be able to provide such students a high-quality inclusive education (Cefai & Spiteri Pizzuto, 2017). Providing opportunities for students with SEBD to be heard provides us with the tools to support them. Students should be seen as sources of knowledge and expertise, able to provide accurate picture of their school life (Cooper, 1996). Studies with SEN students for example show that students primarily need someone to talk, to listen to them and to help resolve their problems (de Boer & Kuijper, 2021). A review of international literature emphasised teachers' personal qualities and skills such as listening to students in the elimination of students' social, emotional and behavioural difficulties (Cooper, 2011; Cooper et al., 2013).

Students with SEBD in Greece suggest that SEBD in classrooms could be interpreted as a synthesis of teachers' and students' social and emotional competences that are manipulable by teachers and can accordingly be modified to achieve desired goals. These data can be used to inform teacher educators and policy makers to identify teacher or students' behaviours and classroom conditions that warrant intervention, and provide additional training and support to classroom teachers, as needed.

Finally, listening to students' voices is the essence of inclusion and democracy (Messiou et al., 2022). By placing students' voice at the core of inclusive process we move a step further to the 'ideal of inclusion' (Kefallinou & Howes, 2002). A democratic education system must focus strongly on the voices of children with difficulties (Herz & Haertel, 2016). With no doubt, the process of empowering students may reveal contradictory and unanticipated messages for schools (Cooper, 2006). On the other hand, if students' voices remain unheard, the discussion on students' rights becomes a humanitarian rhetoric without meaning in practice. Greece has officially adapted the rights-based approach to children's voices but the notion of empowerment and active participation of students with SEBD remains to be adequately represented in research and school practice. In 1989 Paul Cooper first expressed the need for the voices of students with SEBD to be heard, and in 2010 Cefai and Cooper used the term 'students without voices' to underline the need for students with SEBD to be heard. Today, more than three decades later, we still need to raise the voices of students with SEBD both in Greece and internationally.

References

Ainscow, M., & Messiou, K. (2017). Engaging with the views of students to promote inclusion in education. *Journal of Educational Change, 19*(1), 1–17.

Avramidis, E., Avgeri, G., & Strogilos, V. (2018). Social participation and friendship quality of students with special educational needs in regular Greek primary schools. *European Journal of Special Needs Education, 33*(2), 221–234. <https://10.1007/s10447-015-9235-6>.

Bablekou, Z., & Kazi, S. (2016). Intellectual assessment of children and adolescents: The case of Greece. *International Journal of School and Educational Psychology, 4,* 225–230.

Brouzos, A., Vassilopoulos, S., Korfiati, A., & Baourda, V. (2015). Secondary school students' perceptions of their counselling needs in an era of global financial crisis: An exploratory study in Greece. *International Journal of Advanced Counselling, 37,* 168–178. <https://10.1080/08856257.2018.1424779>.

Caslin, M. (2019). 'I have got too much stuff wrong with me'-an exploration of how young people experience the Social, Emotional and Behavioural Difficulties (SEBD) label within the confines of the UK education system. *Emotional and Behavioural Difficulties, 24*(2), 167–180. <https://10.1080/13632752.2019.1587899>.

Cefai, C., & Cooper, P. (2010). Students without voices: The unheard accounts of secondary school students with social, emotional and behavioural difficulties. *European Journal of Special Needs Education, 25*(2), 183–198. <https://10.1080/08856251003658702>.

Cefai, C., & Spiteri Pizzuto, S. A. (2017). Listening to the voices of young children in a nurture class. *Emotional and Behavioural Difficulties, 22*(3), 248–260. <https://10.1080/13632752.2017.1331987>

Christensen, P., & James, A. (2008). *Research with children: Perspectives & practices.* Routledge.

Cook-Sather, A. (2006). Sound, presence, and power: 'Student Voice' in educational research and reform. *Curriculum Inquiry, 36,* 359–390. <https://10.1111/j.1467-873X.2006.00363.x>.

Cooper, P. (1989). *Respite, relationships and re-signification: A study of the effects of residential schooling on children with emotional and behavioural difficulties, with particular reference to the pupils' perspective.* Thesis submitted to the School of Education of the University of Birmingham for the degree of Doctor of Philosophy, UK.

Cooper, P. (1993). Learning from pupils' perspectives. *British Journal of Special Education, 20*(4), 129–133.

Cooper, P. (1996). Pupils as partners: Pupils' contribution to the governance of schools. In K. Jones & T. Charlton (Eds), *Overcoming learning and behaviour difficulties* (pp. 192–207). Routledge.

Cooper, P. (2001). *We can work it out: What works in educating pupils with social emotional and behavioural difficulties: Inclusive practice in mainstream schools.* Routledge/Falmer.

Cooper, P. (2006). John's story: Episode 1 – Understanding SEBD from the inside: The importance of listening to young people. In M. Hunter-Carsch, Y.

Tiknaz, P. Cooper, & R. Sage (Eds), *Handbook of social, emotional and behavioural difficulties* (pp. 16–23). Continuum International Publishing Group.
Cooper, P. (2010). Social, emotional and behavioural difficulties in young people: The challenge for policy makers. *The International Journal of Emotional Education*, 2(1), 4–16.
Cooper, P. (2011). Teacher strategies for effective intervention with students presenting social, emotional and behavioural difficulties: An international review. *European Journal of Special Needs Education*, 26(1), 71–86. <https://10.1080/08856257.2011.543547>.
Cooper, P., Kakos, M., & Jacobs, B. (2011). Best practice models and outcomes in the education of children with social, emotional and behavioural difficulties. *Caise Review*, 1. <https://10.12796/caise-review.2013v1.008>
Davies, J. D. (2005) Voices from the margins: Perceptions of pupils with emotional and behavioural difficulties about their educational experience. In P. Clough, P. P. Garner, J. T. Pardeck, & F. Yeun, F. (Eds), *Handbook of emotional and behavioural difficulties* (pp. 299–316). Sage.
de Boer, A., & Kuijper, S. (2021). Students' voices about the extra educational support they receive in regular education. *European Journal of Special Needs Education*, 36(4), 625–641. <https://10.1080/08856257.2020.1790884>.
de Leeuw, R. R., de Boer, A. A., & Minnaert, A. E. M. G. (2018). Student voices on social exclusion in general primary schools. *European Journal of Special Needs Education*, 33(2), 166–186. <https://10.1080/08856257.2018.1424783>.
European Agency for Special Needs and Inclusive Education. (2020). *Country information for Greece – Legislation and policy* Retrieved from <https://www.european-agency.org/country-information/greece/legislation-and-policy>
Fielding, M., & Bragg, S. (2003). *Students as researchers: Making a difference*. Pearson Publishing.
Flynn, P. (2013). *Authentic listening to student voice: The transformative potential to empower students with social, emotional and behavioural difficulties in mainstream education*. Dublin: TCD (unpublished thesis).
Georgiadi, M., Plexousakis, S., Josi, M., Kourkoutas, E., & Hart, A. (2020). How adolescent students with disabilities and/or complex needs perceive the notion of resilience: A study in Greece and England. *International Journal of Learning, Teaching and Educational Research*, 19(12), 43–69. <https://10.26803/ijlter.19.12.3>.
Government of Greece. (1992). *Official Journal, No. 2101/1992, FEK 192/A/2-12-1992*. Ethniko Typografeio.
Government of Greece. (2012). *Official Journal, No. 4074/2012, FEK 88/A/11-04-2012*. Ethniko Typografeio.

Hall, S. (2010). Supporting mental health and wellbeing at a whole-school level: Listening to and acting upon children's views. *Emotional and Behavioural Difficulties, 15*(4), 323–339. <https://10.1080/13632752.2010.523234>.

Hartas, D., & Geoff, L. (2011). Young people's involvement in service evaluation and decision making. *Emotional and Behavioural Difficulties, 16*(2), 129–143.

Heary, C., & Hennessy, E. (2005). *Developmental changes in children's understanding of psychological problems: A qualitative study*. Paper presented at the Annual Conference of the Psychological Society of Ireland. Galway, Ireland. November.

Herz, B., & Haertel, N. (2016). The pupils voice in different educational settings. *Journal of Research in Special Educational Needs, 16*(1), 1040–1045. <https://10.1111/1471-3802.12249>.

Holdsworth, R., & Blanchard, M. (2006). Unheard voices: Themes emerging from studies of the views about school engagement of young people with high support needs in the area of mental health. *Australian Journal of Guidance and Counselling, 16*(1), 14–28.

Kapi, A., Veltsista, A., Kavadias, G., Lekea,V., & Bakoula, C. (2007). Social determinants of self-reported emotional and behavioral problems in Greek adolescents. *Social Psychiatry and Psychiatric Epidemiology, 42*, 594–598. <https://10.1007/s00127-007-0201-4>.

Kefallinou, A., & Howes, A. (2002). Experiencing 'inclusion': A critical and systemic analysis of young people's voices in English and Greek mainstream secondary schools. *International Journal of Inclusive Education*. <https://10.1080/13603116.2022.2132424>.

Krull, J., Wilbert, J., &. Hennemann, T. (2014). The social and emotional situation of first graders with classroom behavior problems and classroom learning difficulties in inclusive classes. *Learning Disabilities: A Contemporary Journal, 12*(2), 169–190.

Leontopoulou, S., Jimerson, S. R., & Anderson, G. E. (2011). An international exploratory investigation of students' perceptions of stressful life events: Results from Greece, Cyprus and the United States. *School Psychology International, 32*(6), 632–644. <https://10.1177/0143034311403059>.

Lewis, R., & Burman, E. (2008). Providing for student voice in classroom management: Teachers' views. *International Journal of Inclusive Education, 12*(2), 151–167.

Messiou, K., & Hope, M. A. (2015). The danger of subverting students' views in schools. *International Journal of Inclusive Education, 19*(10), 1–13. <https://10.1080/13603116.2015.1024763>.

Messiou, K., Bui, L. T., Ainscow, M., Gasteiger-Klicpera, B., Besic, E., Paleczek, L., ... Echeita, G. (2022). Student diversity and student voice conceptualisations in five European countries: Implications for including all students in schools. *European Educational Research Journal, 21*(2), 355–376.

O' Connor, M., Hodkinson, A., Burton, D., & Torstensson, G. (2011). Pupil voice: Listening to and hearing the educational experiences of young people with behavioural, emotional and social difficulties (BESD). *Emotional and Behavioural Difficulties, 16*(3), 289–302. <https://10.1080/13632752.2011.595095>.

Palikara, O., Castro, S., Gaona, C., & Eirinaki, V. (2018). Capturing the voices of children in the education health and care plans: Are we there yet? *Frontiers In Education, 3*(24). <https://doi.org/10.3389/feduc.2018.00024>

Pappas, M. A., Papoutsi, C., & Drigas, A. (2018). Policies, practices and attitudes toward inclusive education: The case of Greece. *Social Science, 7*, 90–104 <https://doi.org/10.3390/socsci7060090>.

Poulou, M. (2010). The role of Trait Emotional Intelligence and social and emotional skills in students' emotional and behavioural strengths and difficulties: A study of Greek adolescents' perceptions. *The International Journal of Emotional Education, 2*(2), 30–47.

Poulou, M. (2013). Emotionality and social behaviour. *Hellenic Journal of Psychology, 10*(1), 47–60.

Poulou, M. (2014a). The effects on students' emotional and behavioural difficulties of teacher–student interactions, students' social skills and classroom context. *British Educational Research Journal, 40*(6), 986–1004.

Poulou, M. (2014b). How are Trait Emotional Intelligence and social skills related to emotional and behavioural difficulties in adolescents? *Educational Psychology, 34*(3), 354–366. <http://dx.doi.org/10.1080/01443410.2013.785062>.

Poulou, M. (2017). Students' emotional and behavioral difficulties: The role of teachers' social and emotional learning and teacher-student relationships. *The International Journal of Emotional Education, 9*(2), 72–89.

Poulou, M. (2019). Emotion knowledge and social and emotional competence: A preliminary study of preschool and first grade Greek students. *Hellenic Journal of Psychology, 16*, 22–42. <https://doi.org/10.26262/hjp.v16i1.7889>.

Poulou, M. S., & Bassett, H. (2018). Children's emotion and behavior responses to peer provocation and early school adjustment. *Pastoral Care in Education, Special Issue on Mental Health in Schools, 36*(3), 205–222. <https://doi.org/10.1080/02643944.2018.1479351>.

Poulou, M. S., & Cooper, W. P. (2017). Perceptions of sleep duration, patterns and emotional and behavioural difficulties: A study of Greek adolescents. *British Journal of Special Needs Education, 44*(1), 65–94. <https://doi.org/10.1111/1467-8578.12161>.

Poulou, M., & Norwich, B. (2020). Psychological needs, mixed self-perceptions, well-being and emotional and behavioral difficulties: Adolescent students' perceptions. *European Journal of Psychology of Education, 35*, 775–793. <https://doi.org/10.1007/s10212-019-00457-1>.

Poulou, M. S., Grazzani, I., Cavioni, V., Ornaghi, V., Conte, E., Cefai, C., Camilleri, L., & Bartolo, P. (2022a). Changes in students' social and emotional competences following the implementation of a school-based intervention program. *American Journal of Applied Psychology, 11*(5), 122–132. <https://10.11648/j.ajap.20221105.11>

Poulou, M. S., Grazzani, I., Cavioni, V., Ornaghi, V., Conte, E., Cefai, C., Camilleri, L., & Bartolo, P. (2022b). Teachers' and students' changes in social and emotional competences following the implementation of PROMEHS: A European program for Promoting Mental Health at Schools. *Educational Research Application, 7*(1). <https://doi.org/10.29011/2575-7032.100205>.

Rouvali, A., & Riga, V. (2021). Listening to the voice of a pupil with autism spectrum condition in the educational design of a mainstream early years setting. *Education, 3–13, 49*(4), 464–480. <https://10.1080/03004279.2020.173042>.

Rudduck, J., & Flutter, J. (2000). Pupil participation and pupil perspective: 'carving a new order of experience'. *Cambridge Journal of Education, 30*(1), 75–89.

Rudduck, J., & McIntyre, D. (2007). *Improving learning through consulting pupils.* Routledge.

Schwab, S. (2015). Evaluation of a Short version of the Illinois loneliness and social satisfaction scale in a sample of students with and without special educational needs – An empirical study with primary and secondary students in Austria. *British Journal of Special Education, 42*(3), 257–278.

Sellman, E. (2009). Lessons learned: Student voice at a school for pupils experiencing social, emotional and behavioural difficulties. *Emotional and Behavioural Difficulties, 14*(1), 33–48. <https://10.1080/13632750802655687>.

Shallcross, T., Robinson, J., Pace, P., & Tamoutseli, K. (2007). The role of students' voices and their influence on adults in creating more sustainable environments in three schools. *Improving Schools, 10*(1), 72–85. <https://10.1177/1365480207073723>.

Siobhan, M., & Frederickson, N. (2013). Improving pupil referral unit outcomes: Pupil perspectives. *Emotional and Behavioural Difficulties, 18*(4), 407–422. <https://10.1080/13632752.2013.801112>.

Syriopoulou-Delli, C. K. (2010). A historical review of educational policy in Greece for children with pervasive developmental disorders, behavioral difficulties and other special educational needs. *Review of European Studies, 2*(1), 2–14.

Tafa, E., & Manolitsis, G. (2003). Attitudes of Greek parents of typically developing kindergarten children towards inclusive education. *European Journal of Special Needs Education, 18,* 155–171.

Thomsen, P. (2011). Coming to terms with 'Voice.'. In W. Kidd & G. Czerniawski (Eds), *The student voice handbook: Bridging the academic/practitioner divide* (pp. 19–30). Emerald.

UNESCO. (1994). The Salamanca statement and framework for action. *Policy,* June: 50. <https://doi.org/E D –94/WS/1 8>.

UNICEF. (2015). *Incheon declaration.* UNICEF.

Warnock Committee. (1978). *Special educational needs: The Warnock report.* DES.

Whitehurst, T. (2007). Liberating silent voices-perspectives of children with profound and complex learning needs on inclusion. *British Journal of Learning Disabilities, 35,* 55–61. <https://10.1111/j.1468-3156.2006.00405.x>

Zoniou-Sideri, A., Deropoulou-Derou, E., Karagianni, P., & Spandagou, I. (2006). Inclusive discourse in Greece: Strong voices, weak policies. *International Journal of Inclusive Education, 10*(2–3), 279–291. <https://10.1080/13603110500256046>.

COLEEN GILKES-COLLYMORE AND GARRY HORNBY

14 Exploring the Experiences of Mothers of Children with ADHD in the Caribbean

Introduction

The research presented in this chapter was inspired by the work of Paul Cooper, who has published extensively on the topic of Attention Deficit Hyperactivity Disorder (ADHD), particularly on the reality of its existence as a biopsychosocial construct, considering effective interventions in education settings, and focusing on the importance of professionals and parents working collaboratively (e.g. Cooper, 2009, 2010; Cooper & Bilton, 2002; Hughes & Cooper, 2007). In one of his multi-authored research articles, it was found that high quality parent-teacher relationships were the exception, with mothers feeling silenced and criticised (Gwernan-Jones et al., 2015). In this chapter therefore, we present the findings of a study which examined the experience of mothers in parenting children with ADHD and its key role in supporting the learning and positive behaviour of such children.

Background

Attention Deficit Hyperactivity Disorder (ADHD), as defined by the American Psychiatric Association (2013), is still a relatively new research area in the Caribbean, and therefore most of what is known and practiced is grounded in studies conducted abroad. It is considered that children and adolescents with ADHD are under-treated in the Caribbean due to inadequate health care systems, lack of human resources, and poor knowledge of the population with the disorder (Polanczyk et al., 2008).

While many children in the Caribbean are born and raised in two-parent households (Powell, 1986), a high percentage of households are headed by single women (Fyffe, 2021; Stuart, 1996). Female headed households are reported to represent the following proportion of families with children overall: Jamaica: 33.8%; Barbados: 42.9%; Grenada: 45.3% (Massiah, 1982).

Parents of children aged 12 years or younger with ADHD are reported to experience higher parenting stress than do parents of typically developing children (Wong et al., 2018). In fact, a growing body of research confirms that mothers parenting a child with ADHD typically experience high levels of psychological distress and parenting stress (Peters & Jackson, 2009; Theule et al., 2013).

Single mothers in the Caribbean are often the economic providers, primary nurturers and primary caretakers in the home (Bailey et al., 1998). With limited support services available to care for a child with ADHD, the interactions between mother and child have been found to be overwhelmingly negative and marked with increased conflict, especially during adolescence (Climie & Mitchell, 2016; McKee et al., 2004). Impaired family functioning and psychosocial functioning have also been noted, as well as less than ideal parent-school relationships (Johnston & Mash, 2001; Gwernan-Jones et al., 2015).

The current research was needed to understand the social impact of ADHD within the Caribbean context. The researchers were seeking to explore the impact of raising children with ADHD in Barbados, and the wider Caribbean, and to highlight the experiences of mothers, as well as to identify the support needed, that could be addressed through changes in policy, and provision of additional resources. The focus of the study is on the experiences of parenting children with ADHD, parents' experience of the support they have received as a mother parenting a child with ADHD, and the support or help needed in raising a child with ADHD. The purpose of this study was to explore the lived experiences of single mothers raising children with ADHD in Barbados. The three research questions addressed were: *What is your experience of parenting a child with ADHD?*

What is your experience of the support you have received as a mother parenting a child with ADHD? What support or help in raising your child with ADHD would you like to receive?

Method

This research was a qualitative study that relied on human perception and understanding, emphasising personal experience in specific situations (Stake, 2010). Many studies have reported the impacts of ADHD behaviours from the perspectives of parents (Chacko et al., 2009; Papadopoulos, 2021; Wong et al., 2018). However, not much is known about the experiences and perceptions of mothers raising children with ADHD in the Caribbean. In fact, very little research on ADHD has been conducted in the Caribbean (Polanczyk et al., 2008; Youssef et al., 2015) where, because of lack of acknowledgement and awareness of ADHD, it is generally perceived as misbehaviour or laziness on the part of the child, or viewed as a myth (Bowen, 2014; Youssef et al., 2015).

Participants

Participants were selected by convenience sampling from a special education school where the researcher was the principal of the school. The social worker at the school invited fifteen single mothers of children with ADHD to participate in the study. Twelve of the fifteen mothers consented to be involved in the focus groups. All the children had a clinical diagnosis of ADHD. The final sample consisted of ten biological mothers and one foster mother. Mothers' ages ranged from 40 to 60 years with a mean of 45.54. Three out of the eleven mothers lived with extended family members. Nine of the 11 mothers had other children. Only one of the eleven mothers was diagnosed with ADHD herself. Five of the participants were employed; five were unemployed and one worked part-time. Eight of the eleven mothers reported that their highest education level was secondary school. The remaining three mothers received postsecondary education, one of which had a bachelor's degree.

At the time of the interview the children of participants ranged in age from 14 to 21 years with a mean of 16.45 years. They were all male and living with their mothers. Mothers reported that all the children were diagnosed with ADHD, four while at primary school and seven while at secondary school. Diagnosis of ADHD was confirmed by the school social worker. Six out of the eleven children were taking prescribed medication for ADHD; five were receiving occupational therapy; and one was attending drug education and counselling. Eight of the eleven children had at some time been remanded to a correctional facility by the courts. Two of the eleven mothers had sought assistance from an ADHD organisation for help with their children with ADHD.

Data Collection

Three semi-structured focus group interviews and one individual interview with single mothers of adolescents with ADHD were used to collect data. Semi-structured interviews consisted of preformulated questions and prompts used to help participants open up (Ary et al., 2006). The interview questions were designed to address the above research questions. All three focus group interviews were conducted in the conference room at the special school. The first interview consisted of four participants, and second and third interviews consisted of three participants. A separate interview was conducted with one of the mothers who could not attend the focus groups but insisted on taking part in the study.

The focus group interviews were video recorded to allow for repeated revisiting of the data to check emerging themes and ensure that these were true to participants' accounts and enabling reliability checks to be conducted. The focus group interview process followed recommendations from Krueger and Casey (2009) and Pilgrim et al. (2017). Two persons conducted the focus group interviews – the primary researcher and the school social worker. The researcher focused on guiding the discussion, while the social worker observed the reactions of participants and managed the recording of data. A pre-interview warm-up was done to explain the purpose of the study.

The researcher explained the purpose of the study, the three main research questions, and provided an assurance of confidentiality of everything discussed. The researcher then outlined guidelines from Krueger and Casey (2015) with participants before the interviews. Participants were encouraged to listen while others were speaking, respect the views of others and silence phones. Participants were free to have refreshments during the interview. The opening statement used was, 'We would like you to share with us your journey as a mother of a child with ADHD.'

Data Analysis

To ensure accuracy, the researcher transcribed all the interviews. Data analysis was guided by Hyatt's (1986) four sequential stages: familiarisation, selection and ordering, description, and interpretation. The researcher viewed and reviewed video recordings as well as notes from focus group interviews; sorted within the data for patterns, connections and typologies; described what was said in the group in relation to themes identified in the selection and ordering process; and made links to the literature that were identified in the data collected.

Ethical Considerations

The study was approved by the Ministry of Education, Barbados. The ethical guidelines followed were consistent with the University of the West Indies (UWI) International Review Board (IRB) recommendations. Prior to attending focus group interviews, mothers were informed in writing and verbally about the purpose and process of the research, the confidential nature of their contributions, that their participation was voluntary and that they could withdraw at any time without obligation.

Results and Discussion

Eight themes that relate to the experiences of mothers raising children with ADHD emerged from the data: (1) difficulty in managing their child with ADHD's behaviour; (2) impact on relationships with family members and others, (3) ADHD child's school experience – teachers' knowledge, attitudes and behaviour; (4) physical, emotional and social impact on mothers; (5) community views on children's behaviour and mothers' parenting skills; (6) support mothers received in caring for the child with ADHD; (7) support mothers needed for better outcomes; (8) mothers' advice to other parents and the community.

Difficulty in Managing Their Child with ADHD's Behaviour

All mothers in the study expressed that managing their child's behaviour proved difficult and sometimes overwhelming. While some mothers administered medication to regulate their child with ADHD's behaviour, there were concerns about the effects of the medication. Most participants reported resorting to corporal punishment and other physical means to manage behaviour. Sample quotations from mothers follow.

- *I got to play both mother and father too. So I can't make he feel that I weak and he could do what he want.*
- *I used to give real lashes when he do something bad. Talking sometimes they don't listen but if you beat them they would hear.*
- *To be honest I don't care for the medication. It slows them down too much. It doesn't work.*

The research literature supports the finding that mothers raising children with ADHD experience challenging behavioural problems that are demanding, overwhelming and anxiety provoking (Peters & Jackson, 2009). This often results in a 'negative-reactive' pattern from parents more likely having inappropriate parenting strategies, high parental overprotection, and negative parent-child relationships (Gau, 2007).

Regarding medication, Hughes and Cooper (2007) highlight the strengths and limitations, noting that although medication can be a reliable intervention, there are concerns about the development of overreliance on medication and its effects on children. The authors cautioned that medication can never be seen as sufficient treatment in itself as a solution to problems experienced by children suffering with the disorder. Environmental, psychological, and educational interventions are crucial for positive change to occur (Cooper & Bilton, 2002).

Impact on Relationships with Family Members and Others

Participants reported that familial relationships were strained because of their ADHD child's behaviour. In some cases, mothers isolated both themselves and their child from social gatherings to avoid conflict with relatives, believing that no one understood their child. Some quotes illustrating these views follow.

- *I don't really mix with people. I don't hang out.*
- *My mother said don't bring him back. My aunt would say don't bring him back.*
- *When we got certain family functions, I tell myself I ain't going nowhere just so not to get into anything with my family because everybody don't understand he have ADHD.*

The research literature supports the suggestion by Cooper et al. (2019) that ADHD can be viewed as a familial disorder and has been associated with single parenting, as well as low socio-economic and parental educational levels and income (Russell et al., 2016). The increase in conflict between parent and child, family practices and functioning often results in less contact or isolation from extended family members and friends, as well as separation or divorce (Alexander-Roberts, 1995).

ADHD Child's School Experience: Teachers' Knowledge, Attitudes and Behaviour

One of the main concerns expressed by participants was teachers' attitudes and behaviour, and their lack of knowledge and training about ADHD. Participants stated that students with ADHD were being marginalised and victimized by teachers and that their children's academic progress was hampered by teachers in both primary and secondary school. This is illustrated by the following quotations.

- *Well, at primary school I don't think any of the teachers knew anything about ADHD because if he disrupts the class ... they had this one teacher for a whole term would send at the door and he would actually go at the door every day and I didn't know anything about it.*
- *The older teachers would work with him, but the younger teachers told him to get out the class, so he all over the school, he gets into trouble cause he is out of the class.*
- *When they go into secondary school, the teachers are not trained. I don't think that they are trained to deal with children that have a special need like ADHD, dyslexia, that sort of thing.*

Teachers are reported to experience more negative expectations of students with ADHD due to their challenging behaviour, some viewing ADHD as a myth and an excuse for the child's misbehaviour (Ohan et al., 2011). According to Cooper (2009), such negative reactions are based on assumptions that ADHD is biologically determined. Rather, biology is not a sufficient explanation. It is the interplay between genetic make-up, mental health and behaviour, and social and cultural context that determine health related outcomes.

According to Youseff et al. (2015) Caribbean teachers' knowledge about ADHD is insufficient and requires intervention. Cooper (2009) proposes an in depth understanding of the biopsychosocial perspective of education is needed in order to provide effective educational opportunities for children with ADHD.

Physical, Emotional and Social Impact on Mothers

Mothers reported high levels of stress raising their children with ADHD. Shared experiences revealed regret, self-isolation, guilt, self-blame, fear and suicidal ideation. Participants expressed feeling helpless, not knowing enough about ADHD, and of lacking the parenting skills needed to support their children.

- *Before when the school used to call, my heart would race and I couldn't sleep at night until 1 o'clock.*
- *I had to get counselling and was given sleeping pills because I couldn't sleep.*
- *Mentally, physically, it has taken a toll on me. With him I find that I am on edge wondering what he will say and do next.*

The responsibility of caring for a child with ADHD negatively impacts the physical, mental and emotional well-being of caregivers (Balagan & Tarroja, 2020). High levels of stress, depression, anxiety, withdrawal from social groups, and low self-esteem often leads to self-blame for the child's behaviour (Gau, 2007; Wiener et al., 2016). Hughes and Cooper (2007) highlight the importance of active communication between key stakeholders in order to achieve effective interventions at school and home, thereby reducing the above effects.

Community Views on Children's Behaviour and Mothers' Parenting Skills

Mothers felt blamed for their child's behaviour. Their parenting skills were questioned, and many in the community asserted that their children were destined for a life of crime, incarceration and ultimately death by murder.

- *In my district they had a gentleman that used to say oh they are going to get lock up early or somebody is going to kill them.*
- *You ain't a proper mother cause you should beat he.*
- *Bring your leash. Make sure you walk with your leash.*

This present study supports evidence presented in the research literature of parents being confronted with narratives of parental blame and public resistance to the facts surrounding the disorder by professionals and family and community members (Harbourne et al., 2004). This view that ADHD is a myth and an excuse for children's behaviour is based on a lack of understanding of the biopsychosocial perspective of the disorder (Cooper, 2009).

While blame, widespread social stigma and rejection are noted by community members, parents blame themselves for their child's mental health problems and question their own parenting skills (Moses, 2010; Moen et al., 2015; Peters & Jackson, 2009).

Support Received in Caring for the Child with ADHD

Mothers in the study identified school, work and family as the key areas where they felt support was mostly needed. Most participants expressed lack of support in aspects of education, finance and family:

> Education – *Everybody come and take the information and that was it. I always got in contact with people that tell me take him this place and that place.*
>
> Financial – *I get to work late many times and lost my job about three times. He would say "I glad I make you lose your job." I never told my employers about him because they won't understand.*
>
> Family – *My family was not supportive because they would say this boy too hard-ears. Why he ain't like this body and that body.*

Families of children with ADHD encounter many challenges with relatives and the community (McLaughlin & Harrison, 2006; Moen et al., 2015). Support is needed from spouses, relatives, schools, the community and professional providers for improved family relations and to lower the stress level parents experience caring for children with ADHD (Harazni & Alkaissi, 2016; Neff, 2010).

Support Mothers Needed for Better Outcomes

Mothers proposed changes in the educational system to support students with ADHD as well as support for themselves from employers. Closer familial relationships coupled with an ADHD support group was also suggested.

> Education – *It would be good if they had more schools like this (alternative school for at-risk students), or even if the secondary schools had a section or class or division for children who are intelligent but learn differently.*
>
> Work – *I took a one-week vacation and used my vacation days for appointments. Management had a problem with the arrangement, and I left.*
>
> Family – *There wasn't a family to rally around. It was hard on me.*
>
> Support Group – *I feel like you should have groups like how we here sitting down now.*

Participation in support groups is beneficial for parents and caregivers (Chiu et al., 2013). It provides the platform to foster hope while overcoming stigma and isolation. Participants learn about their shared issues and available support services; coping strategies from successful role models to build social support networks; and develop self-confidence to maintain control of situations (Worrall et al., 2018). Noted however, is that for some participants there is an increase in the feeling of being overwhelmed (Heller et al., 1997).

Mothers' Advice to Other Parents and the Community

Mothers in the study were eager to offer advice to other parents and to the community. Examples are presented below.

> Parents – *Children with ADHD cannot do it on their own. They need support. We need to rally around one another.*
>
> Community – *Don't be so quick to judge. Look a little deeper and have an open mind.*

'The voices of the potentially or actually marginalized are a vital element in societies that aspire to social justice' (Hughes & Cooper, 2007, p. 14). Mothers who voice support for their children give encouragement to other parents. Such advocacy influences the development and implementation of policies to ensure that the social, emotional, physical and educational needs of children are met (Wright & Taylor, 2014).

Conclusion

This chapter provides insights into single mothers' experiences of raising a child with ADHD in Barbados and contributes to the existing literature through the description of behaviour management practices, impact on relationships, school experiences, parental well-being, community perceptions, support received, and support needed. The biopsychosocial perspective of ADHD highlighted by Paul Cooper in his writings goes well beyond education and is relevant to many of the findings of this study. 'This helps us (particularly parents and teachers) to make decisions about how we can best help the individual with ADHD by adjusting our behavior towards him or her, and making changes to the environment they experience' (Cooper, 2010, p. 3).

This present study revealed mothers' experience of stress and anxiety from lack of supportive social relationships, conflicts with family members and feelings of incompetence. Cooper and Ideus (2007) encourage collaboration between professionals, parents and children, which the researcher believes can provide single mothers of children with ADHD with the support needed to minimise the negative impact on their mental health. With respect to Paul Cooper's work on ADHD the findings of the current study confirm the critical importance of clarifying our thought process governing behaviour and the consequences this has on the way people think and respond; having effective interventions in education settings and of focusing on working collaboratively with other stakeholders, especially with parents (Cooper & Bilton, 2002; Hughes & Cooper, 2007).

References

Alexander-Roberts, C. (1995). *ADHD and teens: A parent's guide to making it through the tough years*. Taylor.

American Psychiatric Association. (2013). *Diagnostic and statistical manual of mental disorders* (5th edn). American Psychiatric Association.

Ary, D., Jacobs, L. C., & Sorenson, C. (2006). *Introduction to research in education*. Cengage Learning. <http://repository.unmas.ac.id/medias/journal/EBK-00124.pdf>

Bailey, W., Branche, C., & Le Franc, E. (1998). Parenting and socialisation in Caribbean family systems. *Caribbean Dialogue, 4*(1), 21–28. <https://journals.sta.uwi.edu/ojs/index.php/cd/article/view/88>

Balagan, M. M. B., & Tarroja, M. C. H. (2020). Challenges, coping strategies, and needs of mothers with children with attention deficit hyperactivity disorder: Implications for intervention. *Open Journal of Social Sciences, 08*(12), 24–35. <https://doi.org/10.4236/jss.2020.812003>

Bowen, T. (2014). ADHD in the Caribbean. *Caribbean Psychology Today*. <https://caribbeanpsychologytoday.wordpress.com/>

Chacko, A., Wymbs, B. T., Wymbs, F. A., Pelham, W. E., Swanger-Gagne, M. S., Girio, E., Pirvics, L., Herbst, L., Guzzo, J., Phillips, C., & O'Connor, B. (2009). Enhancing traditional behavioral parent training for single mothers of children with ADHD. *Journal of Clinical Child & Adolescent Psychology, 38*(2), 206–218. <https://doi.org/10.1080/15374410802698388>

Chiu, M. Y., Wei, G. F., Lee, S., Choovanichvong, S., & Wong, F. H. (2013). Empowering caregivers: Impact analysis of FamilyLink Education Programme (FLEP) in Hong Kong, Taipei and Bangkok. *International Journal of Social Psychiatry, 59*(1), 28–39. <https://doi.org/10.1177/0020764011423171>

Climie, E. A., & Mitchell, K. (2016). Parent-child relationship and behavior problems in children with ADHD. *International Journal of Developmental Disabilities, 63*(1), 1–9. <https://doi.org/10.1080/20473869.2015.1112498>

Cooper, P. (2009). Like alligators bobbing for poodles? A critical discussion of education, ADHD and biopsychosocial perspective. *Journal of Philosophy of Education, 42*(3–4), 457–474. <https://doi.org/10.1111/j.1467-9752.2008.00657.x>

Cooper, P. (2010). ADHD: Not just biology or environment. ADHD is a biopsychosocial issue *Psychology Today*. <https://www.psychologytoday.com/nz/blog/the-innovative-learner/201010/adhd-not-just-biology-or-environment>

Cooper, P., & Bilton, K. M. (2002). *Attention deficit hyperactivity disorder: A practical guide for teachers* (2nd edn). Routledge. <https://doi.org/10.4324/9780203462331>

Cooper, P., & Ideus, K. (2007). Is attention deficit hyperactivity a Trojan horse? *Support for Learning, 10*(1), 29–34. <https://doi.org/10.1111/j.1467-9604.1995.tb00007.x>.

Cooper, P., Lai, C., Poon, C., Luan, X., Chong, S., & Ng, K. (2019). *Guidebook for supporting students with emotional and behavioural difficulties.* The Education University of Hong Kong.

Fyffe, D. N. (2021). Caribbean family diversity: The factors responsible for such family diversity. *Jamaica Pen.* <https://theislandjournal.com/2021/04/15/jamaican-lifestyle-caribbean-family-diversity-part-2/>

Gau, S. S. (2007). Parental and family factors for attention-deficit hyperactivity disorder in Taiwanese children. *Australian and New Zealand Journal of Psychiatry, 41,* 688–696. <https://doi.org/10.1080/00048670701449018>.

Gwernan-Jones, R. C., Moore, D. A., Garside, R., Richardson, M., Thompson-Coon, J., Rogers, M., ... Forde, T. J. (2015). ADHD, parent perspectives and parent teacher relationships: Grounds for conflict. *British Journal of Special Education, 42*(3). <https://doi.org/10.1111/1467-8578.12087>.

Harazni, L., & Alkaissi, A. (2016). The experience of mothers and teachers of attention deficit/hyperactivity disorder children, and their management practices for the behaviors of the child: A descriptive phenomenological study. *Journal of Education and Practice, 7*(6), 1–21.

Harbourne, A., Wolpert, M., & Clare L. (2004). Making sense of ADHD: A battle for understanding? Parents' views of their children being diagnosed with ADHD. *Clinical Child Psychology and Psychiatry 9,* 327–339.

Heller, T., Roccoforte, J. A., Hsieh, K., Cook, J. A., & Pickett, S. A. (1997). Benefits of support groups for families of adults with severe mental illness. *American Journal of Orthopsychiatry, 67*(2), 187–198. <https://doi.org/10.1037/h0080222>.

Hughes, L., & Cooper, P. (2007). *The ADHD experience.* SAGE. <https://doi.org/10.4135/9781446212998>.

Hyatt, J. (1986). Analysis of qualitative data. In J. Ritchie & W. Sykes (Eds), *Advanced workshop in applied qualitative research* (pp. 32–39). Social and Community Planning Research.

Johnston, C., & Mash, E. J. (2001). Families of children with attention-deficit/hyperactivity disorder: Review and recommendations for future research. *Clinical Child and Family Psychology Review, 4*(3), 183–207. <https://doi.org/101023/a:1017592030434>.

Krueger, R., & Casey, M. (2009). *Focus groups: A practical guide for applied research* (4th edn). Sage.

Krueger, R. A., & Casey, M. A. (2015). *Handbook of practical program evaluation* (4th edn). Wiley. <https://doi.org/10.1002/9781119171386.ch.20>.

Massiah, J. (1982). Female-headed households and employment in the Caribbean. *Women's Studies International*,*2*, 7–16. <http//www.jstor.org/stable/40213425>

McKee, T. E., Harvey, E., Danforth, J. S., Ulaszek, W. R., & Friedman, J. L. (2004). The relation between parental coping styles and parent-child interactions before and after treatment for children with ADHD and oppositional behavior. *Journal of Clinical Child and Adolescent Psychology*, *33*(1), 158–168. <https://doi.org/10.1207/S15374424JCCP3301_15>.

McLaughlin, D. P., & Harrison, C. A. (2006). Parenting practices of mothers of children with ADHD: The role of maternal and child factors. *Child and Adolescent Mental Health*, *11*(2), 82–88. <https://doi.org/10.1111/j.1475-3588.2005.00382.x>.

Moen, Ø. L., Hedelin, B., & Hall-Lord, M. L. (2015). Parental perception of family functioning in everyday life with a child with ADHD. *Scandinavian Journal of Public Health*, *43*(1), 1–8. <https://doi.org/10 1177/1403494814559803>.

Moses, T. (2010). Exploring parents' self-blame in relation to adolescents' mental disorders. *Family Relations: An Interdisciplinary Journal of Applied Family Studies*, *59*(2), 103–120. <https://doi.org/10.1111/j.1741-3729.2010.00589.x>

Neff, P. E. (2010). Fathering an ADHD child: An examination of paternal well-being and social support. *Sociological Inquiry*, *80*(4), 531–533. <https://doi.org/10.1111/j.1475-682x.2010.00348.x>.

Ohan, J. L., Visser, T. A., Strain, M. C., & Allen, L. (2011). Teachers' and education students' perceptions of and reactions to children with and without the diagnostic label 'ADHD'. *Journal of School Psychology*, *49*(1), 81–105. <https://doi.org/10.1016/j.jsp.2010.10.001>.

Papadopoulos, D. (2021). Mothers' experiences and challenges raising a child with autism spectrum disorder: A qualitative study. *Brain Sciences*, *11*, 309. <https//doi.org/10.3390/brainsci11030309>.

Peters, K., & Jackson, D. (2009). Mothers' experiences of parenting a child with attention deficit hyperactivity disorder. *Journal of Advanced Nursing*, *65*(1), 62–71. <https://doi.org/10.1111/j.1365-2648.2008.04853.x>.

Pilgrim, M., Hornby, G., & Macfarlane, S. (2017). Enablers and barriers to developing competencies in a blended learning programme for specialist teachers in New Zealand. *Educational Review*, *70*(5), 548–564.

Polanczyk, G., Rohde, L. A., Szobot, C., Schmitz, M., Montiel-Nava, C., & Bauermeister, J. J. (2008). ADHD treatment in Latin America and the

Caribbean. *Journal of the American Academy of Child & Adolescent Psychiatry*, 47, 721–722.

Powell, D. (1986). Caribbean women and their response to familial experiences. *Social and Economic Studies*, 35(2), 83–130. <http:www.jstor.org/stable/27862840>.

Russell, A. E., Ford, T., Williams, R., & Russell, G. (2016). The association between socioeconomic disadvantage and attention deficit/hyperactivity disorder (ADHD): A systematic review. *Child Psychiatry and Human Development*, 47(3), 440–458. <https://doi.org/10.1007/s10578-015-0578-3>.

Stake, R. (2010). *Qualitative research: Studying how things work.* Guilford.

Stuart, S. (1996). Female-headed families: A comparative perspective of the Caribbean and the developed world. *Gender and Development* 4(2), 28–34. <https://doi.org/10.1080/741922017>.

Theule, J., Wiener, J., Tannock, R., & Jenkins, J. M. (2013). Parenting stress in families of children with ADHD: A meta-analysis. *Journal of Emotional and Behavioral Disorders*, 21(1), 3–17. <https://doi.org/10.1177/1063426610387433>.

Wiener, J., Biondic, D., Grimbos, T., & Herbert, M. (2016). Parenting stress of parents of adolescents with attention-deficit hyperactivity disorder. *Journal of Abnormal Child Psychology*, 44(3), 561–574.

Wong, I., Hawes, D. J., Clarke, S. D., Kohn, M. R., & Dar-Nimrod (2018). Perceptions of ADHD among diagnosed children and their parents: A systematic review using the common-sense model of illness representations. *Clinical Child and Family Psychology Review*, 21(3). <https://doi.org/10.1007/s10567-017-0245-2>.

Worrall, H., Schweizer, R., Marks, E., Yuan, L., Lloyd, C., & Ramjan, R. (2018). The effectiveness of support groups: A literature review. *Mental Health and Social Inclusion*, 22(2), 85–93. <https://doi.org/10.1108/MHSI-12-2017-0055>.

Wright, A. C., & Taylor, S. (2014). Advocacy by parents of young children with special needs: Activities, processes, and perceived effectiveness. *Journal of Social Service Research*, 40(5), 1–15. <https://doi.org/10.1080/01488376.2014.896850>.

Youssef, M. K., Hutchinson, G., & Youssef, F. F. (2015). Knowledge of and attitudes toward ADHD among teachers: Insights from a Caribbean nation. *SAGE Open*, 5(1). <https://doi.org/10.1177/2158244014566761>.

Notes on Contributors

CORINNA BARKER, MA, is a teacher at Greenleaf Primary School, London, UK and has also worked in an inner-city school in Leeds. The research reported in her chapter comes from her Masters' thesis carried out at Liverpool Hope University. She has a passion for working creatively with young children through art, dance, drama and story, and continues to explore the ways in which early experiences in the family influence later social and emotional development across the lifespan.

CARMEL BORG, PhD, is Head of the Department of Arts, Open Communities and Adult Education, at the Faculty of Education, University of Malta. He lectures in sociology of education; curriculum studies; critical pedagogy; adult education for community development; and parental involvement in education. He is the author, co-author, and editor of twenty books, as well as academic papers and chapters in books that explore the relationship between education, democracy, and social justice. Borg is the editor of the Malta Review of Educational Research (MRER), Postcolonial Directions in Education (PDS), and the Education Research Monograph Series (ERMS). Borg was appointed to Malta's National Order of Merit in December 2022.

VALERIA CAVIONI, PhD, is a psychologist, psychotherapist, and a researcher in developmental and educational psychology at the University of Foggia, in Italy. Her main research interests include the design, implementation, and evaluation of school-based programs to support mental health, social and emotional learning as well as the resilience of students and teachers. She has been involved in several national and international projects and she collaborated with the European Commission, UNESCO, and OECD. She authored various scientific publications, books, and reports for policymakers.

CARMEL CEFAI, PhD, FBPS, is the Director of the Centre for Resilience and Socio-emotional Health, and Professor at the Department of Psychology, at the University of Malta. He is Honorary Chair of the European Network for Social and Emotional Competence, joint founding editor of the International Journal of Emotional Education, and a member of the European Commission Network of Experts on Social Aspects of Education and Training. He has led various local, national, European, and international research projects in social and emotional learning, mental health in schools, children's voices, and resilience and wellbeing in children and young people. He has published extensively with numerous books, research reports, journal papers and book chapters.

DAVID COLLEY, PhD, leads the Post Graduate Diploma in Social Emotional and Mental Health Difficulties at Oxford Brookes University (UK) and is Research Associate with the Mulberry Bush Organisation (UK). When completing his PhD, David was supervised by Professor Cooper with whom he later co-edited the key Teacher Training text 'Attachment and Emotional Development in the Classroom'. David's current research is investigating the impact of whole school nurturing practices in both primary and secondary school settings.

PAUL COOPER, PhD, CPsychol, FBPsS, is Emeritus Professor at Brunel University, London, and Visiting Professor at the University of Malta. He has also held research and academic posts at: the Universities of Birmingham, Oxford, Cambridge, Leicester, and the Hong Kong Institute of Education (now The Hong Kong University of Education). He has been Visiting Professor at universities in Japan, Australia, Taiwan and the USA. His research and publications, spanning forty years, have focused on: social, emotional and behaviour difficulties in schools; effective teaching and learning with particular attention to the needs of students with social and emotional difficulties, and the biopsychosocial paradigm. He has produced over 200 publications, including 30 books, and has presented at many conferences throughout the world.

Notes on Contributors

HELEN COWIE, PhD, is a Fellow of the British Psychological Society and a Chartered Counselling Psychologist. She has published widely on anti-bullying interventions at school and university and on the emotional health and wellbeing of children, to include A School for Everyone by Helen Cowie|Hachette UK a book of stories for children to celebrate diversity and promote inclusivity. In 2020 the University of Malta published her Monograph Helen Cowie Peer Support in School final Online. pdf (um.edu.mt) *Peer Support in Schools*. In 2023 Routledge published *Cyberbullying and Online Harms: From Community to Campus*, co-authored by her with Carrie-Anne Myers Cyberbullying and Online Harms: Preventions and Interventions from Com (<routledge.com>).

PAUL DOWNES, PhD, is Director of the Educational Disadvantage Centre, Professor of Education (Psychology), Institute of Education, Dublin City University. He has been involved in various expert advisory roles for the European Commission in areas of social inequalities, lifelong learning, second chance education, school governance and early school leaving. He has over 100 publications of books, articles in international peer-reviewed journals and book chapters in areas of education, psychology, philosophy, law, anthropology and social policy. His books include *Reconstructing agency in developmental and educational psychology: Inclusive Systems as Concentric Space, Concentric Space as a Life Principle Beyond Schopenhauer, Nietzsche and Ricoeur: Inclusion of the Other* and *The Primordial Dance: Diametric and Concentric Spaces in the Unconscious World*.

CHRIS FORLIN, PhD, is a Professorial Research Fellow at the University of Notre Dame Australia. She has extensive consultancy, research, and publications over the past 40 + years with a strong focus on equity and diversity; inclusive education; change paradigms in education; systemic support for children and youth with disabilities; education policy and practice; along with curricula and pedagogy for teacher education, with innovative research in working with systems, governments, and schools to establish sustainable inclusive education.

COLEEN DILKES-COLLYMORE, MA, has been a Special Needs educator in Barbados for the past twenty-seven years. She is currently a principal at a primary school; and is the former Programme Director of an alternative school for at-risk children. Coleen attained her Bachelor of Education (BEd) degree in Special Education from Mount Saint Vincent University, and a Master of Education degree in Literacy Studies at the University of the West Indies, Cave Hill. She is presently pursuing a Doctor of Philosophy (PhD) degree at the same university. She is the recipient of the prestigious Royal Fidelity National Distinguished Teacher Award (2014).

MICHALIS KAKOS, PhD, joined Leeds Beckett University in September 2013. Previously he was leading the University of Leicester Postgraduate Certificate Course in Citizenship Education. He has also held research fellowships in the Centre for Citizenship and Human Rights Education (CCHRE), University of Leeds, and in the Centre for Research in Inclusion and Diversity (CREID), University of Edinburgh. Michalis's research and teaching experience cover the areas of citizenship and intercultural education, inclusive education and special educational needs. The aspect of schooling that Michalis is particularly interested in is the interaction between students and teachers and its role in young people's self-concept and socialisation.

COLLEEN MCLAUGHLIN, PhD, Professor Emerita at the University of Cambridge, is an independent researcher and developer. She held various positions: at Cambridge, Special Advisor to the VC, the Director of Education Innovation at the Faculty of Education and Deputy Head of Faculty; and Head of Department at the University of Sussex. She has worked with governments on education reform in many international contexts. Her interests are mental health and the school's role, education reform, teacher development, and school-university research partnerships.

BRAHM NORWICH, PhD, is Professor of Educational Psychology and Special Educational Needs at the School of Education, University of Exeter, and previously Professor of Special Needs Education at the Institute of Education, University of London. He has worked as a teacher, a professional educational psychologist, lecturer, and researcher. In addition to many academic research papers, he has written about: Special needs a new look. with Mary Warnock (Continuum Books, 2010); Experiencing special educational needs; lessons for practice (Open University Press 2017) and Addressing tensions and dilemmas in inclusive education; resolving democratically (Routledge, 2024).

MARIA POULOU, PhD, is an Associate Professor in Educational Psychology at the University of Patras, Greece. Her work focuses on classroom management, students' emotional and behavioural difficulties, mental health at schools, and teachers' professional development. She has published numerous papers and book chapters in English and in Greek. She is a Fellow of International and National Associations, reviewer for refereed international journals, and National and International grant agencies. She has received grants from the Greek Foundation, the International School Psychology Association, and the Fulbright Foundation.

GIUSI ANTONIA TOTO, PhD, is full professor of Didactics and Special Pedagogy at the Department of Humanities at the University of Foggia, Italy, where she coordinates the Learning Science Hub, a multidisciplinary research centre whose activities focus on innovation in teaching and learning processes from an inclusive perspective. She is the coordinator of the course of study in Psychological Sciences and Techniques, and Rector's Delegate for Teacher Training and Continuing Education.

KATE WINCHESTER, PhD, is a senior lecturer in the School of Education at Notre Dame University Australia, Sydney campus. Her areas of research are in arts education, student engagement and learning, and creativity. Kate has had teaching experience in educational contexts in Australia and the UK at primary and tertiary levels. Kate began working in schools as an Arts facilitator in disadvantaged schools in the United Kingdom. She is currently a facilitator and lecturer who is passionate about inspiring active positive change, social justice, self-reflection, creativity, and authentic learning.

SU QIONG XU, PhD, is Associate Professor of Education at the School of Education, Chongqing Normal University, Chongqing, Shapingba, China. She is also affiliated at the Chongqing Key Laboratory of Psychological Diagnosis and Education Technology for Children with Special Needs and the School of Education, University of Saint Joseph, Macao, China. She has numerous publications in international journals with a particular focus on inclusive education.

Index

Action Knowledge 21–22
ADHD and biopsychosocial perspective 7, 54–55, 55–58
ADHD and parenting 9, 229–231, 231–240
Arts based pedagogy 9, 178–179

Biopsychosocial perspective
    Biopsychosocial perspective of ADHD 7, 54–55, 55–58
    Biopsychosocial perspective of SEND 4, 54–55
    Biopsychosocial perspective and psychological development 77–80
    Biopsychosocial perspective and social model 58–61
Boxall Profile 62, 132

Cooper, P. 3–11, 13, 22, 23, 25, 27, 28, 29, 31, 35, 46, 49, 53–65, 67–68, 72–78, 81, 82, 85–86, 101–102, 105–106, 109–110, 118, 121, 122, 123, 127–138, 139–140, 151, 153, 167, 169, 175, 177, 197–199, 206, 209, 211, 214–216, 218, 220–221, 222–223, 225, 229, 235–238, 240, 241–242

Diametric and Concentric Spatial Systems 69–71

Exclusion 9, 199–202

Fair Go Programme (FOG) 179–185
Father-child attachment 8, 154–156

Group membership 42–43

Hargreaves, D. 15–18, 19, 23, 32

Identity 7, 40–42, 47–48
Inclusion 7–8, 61–64, 199
    Inclusion and engagement 61–64
    Inclusion and relational spaces 7, 67–68
    Inclusion as differing 46–47
    Inclusive education 7, 109–110
Initial teacher education 7, 85–87, 100–103, 211–213
Interventions for SEBD 9, 139, 166, 175, 197

Mead, M. 16, 39
Mental health in school 202–207
Milani, Don Lorenzo 141

Nurture groups
    Attachment 128, 166
    Development 5, 127–129
    Effectiveness 129–132
    Emancipatory nurturing in education 139–140
    Emancipatory nurture groups 139, 143–145
    Nurturing cities 132–134
    Nurturing presence 91
    Principles 130, 167
    Relational spaces 72

Optimal Distinctiveness Theory 44–45
Other, the 40–42

Out of school children 9, 199–202

SEBD
    Ecosystemic perspective 3–4
    SEBD and disengagement 175–176
    SEBD and inclusion 62–64
    SEBD and special schools 23, 25–27
    SEBD and student voices 215–221
Social and emotional education 6, 10, 67
    Commodification of 75–77
Social and emotional learning 178
Social and emotional wellbeing 8, 10
Spatial framework in education 7, 67–68, 77–82

Special education teachers 8, 86–87
Special education reforms 111–115, 116–121
Student disengagement 9, 175–176
Student engagement 177, 185–189
Student voices 9, 73–74, 211–214
    Student voice and SEBD 215–221
Symbolic Interactionist approach 16, 36–39

Teacher-student relationship 86
Transformative educators 148–150

Upton, G. 28–29

www.ingramcontent.com/pod-product-compliance
Ingram Content Group UK Ltd.
Pitfield, Milton Keynes, MK11 3LW, UK
UKHW021706160125
4146UKWH00033B/843